SPROUTS

Live Well with Living Foods

IAN GIESBRECHT

MICROCOSM PUBLISHING

PORTLAND, OREGON

SPROUTS: LIVE WELL WITH LIVING FOODS

Edited by Elly Blue & Taylor Hurley

Cover & design by Meggyn Pomerleau

This edition first published September 13, 2016

Microcosm Publishing

2752 N Williams Ave.

Portland, OR 97227

www.microcosmpublishing.com

ISBN 978-1-62106-491-6

Distributed by Legato / Perseus Books Group and Turnaround, U.K.

Printed on post-consumer paper in the U.S.

Library of Congress Cataloging-in-Publication Data

Names: Giesbrecht, Ian.

Title: Sprouts : live well with living foods / by Ian Giesbrecht.

Description: First edition. | Portland, Oregon : Microcosm Publishing, 2016.

Identifiers: LCCN 2015048989 (print) | LCCN 2016016865 (ebook) | ISBN 9781621064916 (pbk.) | ISBN 9781621064367 (pdf) | ISBN 9781621063537 (epub) | ISBN 9781621062653 (mobi)

Subjects: LCSH: Sprouts.

Classification: LCC SB324.53 .G54 2016 (print) | LCC SB324.53 (ebook) | DDC 641.6/536--dc23

LC record available at https://lccn.loc.gov/2015048989

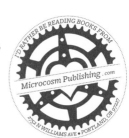

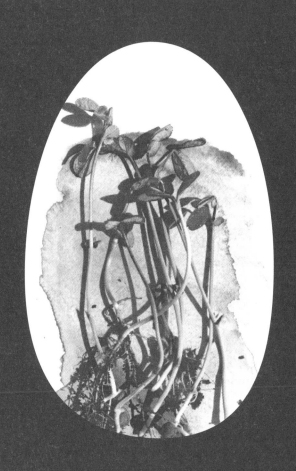

TABLE OF

CONTENTS

INTRODUCTION

In today's swamp of new-age dieting fads and fancy food modifiers, it is often difficult to find simple, accessible ways to eat right. This manual is for the health-conscious and the mindful who are looking for the link between taking responsibility for their personal health and for their surrounding environment. In this book, I introduce the benefits, concepts, theories and practice of sprouting as part of a holistic health strategy. I will teach you all about sprouting and how to incorporate it naturally into your life. Bringing the yesterday into tomorrow, this manual offers ideas and advice for a more vibrant life through sprouting.

SPROUTING OFFERS:

1. An opportunity to empower yourself and produce local, higher-energy food

2. An economical and accessible food source

3. A source of chlorophyll to oxygenate and cleanse the blood

4. A good way to strengthen the immune system

5. A host of phytochemicals and vitamins to protect the body

6. High-quality nourishment, including digestible protein and healthy fats

7. Support for cellular regeneration

8. Alkalization of the body, discouraging pathogens and disease

Within these pages, I hope to provide the seeds of inspiration by offering an overview of the health benefits, growing methods, and recipes of sprouting.

My goal is ultimately to germinate growth within the life of the reader.

This work is an invitation to connect more deeply with our life cycles, and to be reminded of the miracles of life. You'll find information on specific constituents that promote and preserve human (and animal) health, instructions on growing a variety of sprouts, ideas and recipes for using sprouts, and some resources to get you started. My hope is to get you wanting to sprout and to equip you to do so.

The sacred unfolding into life a seed undertakes as it sprouts is a reminder of our potential for growth and regeneration. The steps are simple and the relationship is life long. Sprouting is a valuable part of an effective wellness strategy. To begin it requires only a subtle shift in approach and an intentional sense of awareness.

WHAT IS FOOD?

Within each of us lies an opportunity for vitality—a chance to realize our ultimate potential by harmonizing with our surroundings. We are sacred beings filled with unlimited power for growth. The metabolic processes responsible for the miracle that are our bodies rely on sunlight, which is the ultimate energy source for life on earth. As humans, we depend highly on plants for energy as well. Realizing and respecting this dependence encourages the fostering of relationships among humans and other life forms and cycles.

Our entire existence hinges on harnessing and incorporating the energy from one of the many forms it may take. The stage of life at which we consume molecules is monumentally important; these are the molecules that will build the cells that become our bodies. This is a simple but often overlooked reality in the modern world.

Current food systems are not geared towards health, but rather efficiency and consistency. It seems that we are playing a global game of roulette by splicing genes from different species through genetic modification, without due course for experimentation. We forget what natural food essentially is when crops are bred in a laboratory, fed with synthesized nutrients, and then grown with harmful chemicals in abused and degraded soil. To add insult to injury, much of the "fresh" produce we purchase and enjoy is flown in from around the globe, and usually arrives on our plates several days (or more) after harvest. It's also sprayed with numerous agents to retard mold and pests, or to increase ripening. Even "organic" has become a mainstream buzzword, not always connected to the biological life of the food it describes.

Furthermore, many of the foods we eat are stripped of their nutrients in the act of processing and then have synthesized nutrients added later, along with innumerable additives such as coloring, preservatives, and other food-like substances. The ever-increasing rates of industrial health conditions such as diabetes, obesity, and heart disease and cardiovascular disorders have been directly linked to overconsumption of these edible food-like substances, unhealthy fats, and refined foods. This gives the acronym SAD (Standard American Diet) a whole new meaning.

This global food system is inherently dependent on machines that run on, and products that are made of, fossil fuels. Store-bought "organic" spinach was most likely brought to you in no small part by petroleum. Re-localizing and adjusting the timeframe of our food systems is an effective and comprehensive way to address the myriad of problems faced by the human race and other creatures of the earth.

This may seem an overwhelming task for "them"—the policy makers, the farmers, the food producers, and large companies—to take on. Yet large shifts can be made one person and one decision at a time. One decision leads to another as one more bit of inspiration makes waves. It's never too late to make changes. No act is too small to make a big difference.

>> *"When diet is wrong, medicine is of no use.* <<
When diet is correct, medicine is of no need"
-Ayurvedic proverb

RETURNING SIMPLY TO SOURCE

In a world where buzzwords and fad diets are floating in the collective consciousness, it takes wading through a ton of information just to make informed food choices. Contradictions within scientific research, freshly discovered compounds, and "new" superfoods, combined with our fanaticism, can make eating for health a real challenge.

This is not the place to discuss the hippest or most effective diet, nor is it the place to denounce or criticize food choices. My intention is simply to offer details on how to be more engaged in the process of growth and nourishment through sprouting.

Our industrial food systems replace personal relationships for mechanical advantage. We live in a globalized economy where we eat apples from Chile, cacao (usually as chocolate) from Ghana, goji berries from China, and lettuce from California, all the while living amongst farmers who are unable to eat the food they grow for cows. The food industry is not going to change overnight, even with one giant act towards shifting it. To enable change, we need to start small and plan for success, especially if we continue to engage in consuming living or once-living beings.

Sprouting is the simplest of things, allowing a seed to do what it is meant to do—grow. Sprouting offers a window into the miraculous world of plant life, personal empowerment, and the wonders of watching things grow. It is a gateway and an invitation to another way of perceiving and engaging with the life of plants, as well as your personal food life. This small step may be the first of many on your way to a more committed and involved relationship with life.

Almost all food once began as a seed. For example, the largest walnut tree began as a seed. The mighty alfalfa with the potential to send its roots down 49 ft (15 m) had its humble beginnings as a seed. And even the animals we raise for meat ate food that originated as seeds. Returning to this is so simple, yet often overlooked in most of today's food system, with the exception of a few conciliatory alfalfa sprouts served at delis, or the mung-bean sprouts in Asian stir-fries.

Sprouting can be about simply feeling in touch with your food, embarking on a therapeutic diet, detoxifying, boosting your immunity, saving money, or reducing your carbon food footprint. Sprouting is not a new fad, nor is it complex or overly time-consuming. It's easy enough even for children to do, and can benefit everyone by offering a meaningful and immediate connection to healthcare and diet.

Take control of your life source with compassionate awareness and informed action. Engage in the intimacies of lifecycles, and revel in all the joys experienced through the growth process of safe and sustainable food systems on a community and global level. Sprouts can be grown anywhere all year round; the seeds store and ship easily and can be transformed into vital food using local energy and resources like water, sun, air, and earth. Through sprouting, the possibility exists to take some strain off the globalized food system.

Soak up the sun. Spread the seeds. Harvest and be merry. Tread lightly on our Earth Mother and there shall be overflowing abundance. Unify to cultivate wellness and bring the most radiantly alive energy source to your body.

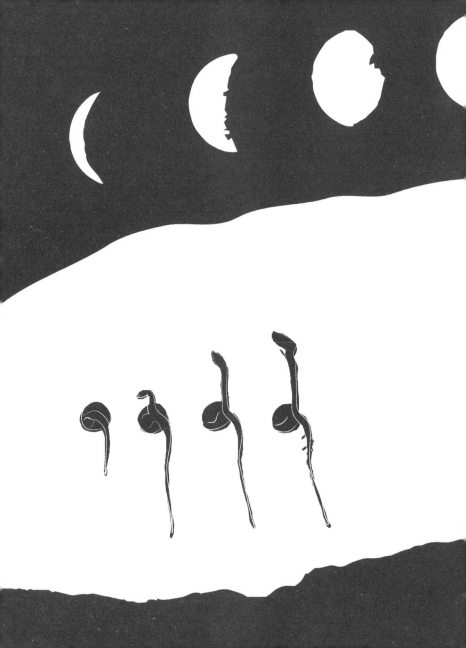

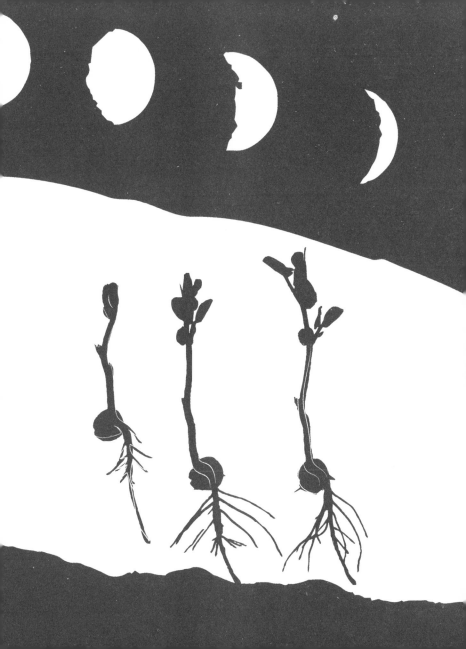

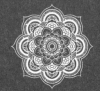

THE SCIENCE OF SPROUTING

Sprouts are very young, living seeds—somewhere between seed and plant. Sprouting entails the beginning stages of life for a seed. It is through the miraculous process of germination that begins a series of changes a dormant seed goes through en route to becoming a plant. By offering seeds adequate moisture and heat, they are activated and begin to come alive.

A sprout prepares itself for new life by sending a radicle (seed or embryonic root) downward to anchor itself in the soil, while sending a plumule (seed or embryonic shoot) upward to photosynthesize in the sunlight. At this early sprout stage, the cotyledons (seed or embryonic leaves) begin to unfurl and take in light for chlorophyll production.

This process can be achieved with or without a medium (see Medium Options, page 69), depending on the seed and the desired outcome. Seeds that are grown with media are know as microgreens. Like sprouts, microgreens are eaten at the cotyledon stage, before true leaves emerge—although some crops may be suited to eat after the true leaves emerge.

There is alchemy underway as the seed germinates, demonstrated by the marked improvement in the amino acid composition, the quality and quantity of vitamins, and the overall digestibility. Vitamins and enzymes are very perishable and deteriorate rapidly once produce is harvested (more details on enzymes and vitamins can be found later in this chapter). The most effective delivery system for these sensitive nutrients is eating food as a living plant source. Sprouts offer this and can be grown in every home or kitchen.

Modern research validates the use of sprouting in high-quality nutrition. For instance, while conducting research at Cornell University in the 1940s, renowned biochemical nutritionist Dr. Clive McCay was one of the first scientists to prove that sprouts had nutritional value. He described sprouts in glowing terms: "A live vegetable that will grow in any climate, rival meat in nutritional value (and tomatoes in vitamin C), mature in three to five days, may be planted any day of the year, require neither soil nor sunshine and can be eaten raw."

This is not new knowledge. Sprouting has played an integral role in numerous cultures for millennia. Edward Howell, a widely respected enzyme expert and author of *Enzyme Nutrition*, states that the majority of grains eaten historically around the globe before industrial agriculture became common were likely at least partially germinated. Germination techniques were and are used by makers of bulgur in the Middle East, as well as in the making of beer through harnessing the potential of sprouting in the malting process. Citing a more extreme example, Europeans developed vitamin supplements using bean sprouts to help sailors avoid scurvy outbreaks during long sea voyages when fresh foods were scarce. For 5,000 years, the Chinese have been growing and eating mung bean and soybean sprouts to ensure adequate vitamin C on sea voyages, and to aid digestion, reduce inflammation, and calm the nerves. Sprouting was also employed by ancient Jewish mystics known as the Essenes, who made bread from living grains and legumes.

GERMINATION: SUPPORTING OUR DIGESTION & ASSIMILATION

The act of germination is a marvel in itself; it essentially activates seeds, waking them up from a dormant state by soaking them in water. This simplifies nutrients into manageable, bite-size pieces. The germination process transforms stored nutrients into bioavailable vitamins, minerals, proteins, and fats that are easily digested and assimilated in the body. In their dormant forms, these reserve nutrients are stable (good for the seed) but not nutritionally accessible to us. As enzyme activity increases, so does metabolic movement. Complex carbohydrates, or starches, are broken down to simple sugars while proteins are broken down to amino acids. These nutrients are transformed through sprouting to become much more bioavailable, allowing the seeds to do a large part of the digestive work for our bodies.

>> *"Natural forces within us are the true healers of disease."* <<
·Hippocrates

BIOACTIVE CATALYSTS: LIFESOURCE NUTRITION

Sprouting is the process that begins most plant life on earth. Given the correct conditions, such as adequate heat and moisture, a seed is transformed through germination from a dense source of stored energy into an active being. As the plant is awakened and the growth process begins, not only are the dormant macronutrients (proteins, fats, and carbohydrates) broken down, but micronutrients (vitamins, minerals, polyphenols, etc.) are activated, increasing in both quantity and availability.

Food guides tell us to follow the Recommended Daily Intake (RDI), but growing research shows that good nutrition is not only about simply getting the vitamins, carbohydrates, and other nutrients, but it's also about understanding where they come from and in what form. How are we connected to and dependent on our environment? A more practical approach than simply reading the RDI is to focus on the bio-availability of foods that we eat. By knowing the basics of this intricate concept, we can support our own body's connection to other life forms through sprouting our food.

When consumed, sprouts offer a cache of accessible vitamins, minerals, antioxidants, anti-carcinogens, and protein, as well as beneficial chlorophyll. The seeds from which the young plant grows are storehouses of nutrients, designed to give the new plant fuel for growth and repair. By eating the germinating seeds and their young shoots, we are able to fully utilize the abundant life and growth contained within them.

ANTIOXIDANTS: THE GUARDIANS OF DNA

Antioxidants are well known for their ability to prevent cellular damage. They were originally an evolutionary trait developed to protect plants from the by-products of photosynthesis and have received significant scientific inquiry in recent years.

As modern humans, we are exposed to a number of free radicals from a wide variety of sources ranging from pollution, chemicals in our water, or improperly prepared or contaminated food. This adds to the burden of the regular effects of aging.

Free radicals are unstable molecules with unpaired electrons; they can be very stressful on the body due to their ability to damage cellular tissue. They are neutralized by antioxidants that donate an electron to pair with the unstable free radical. Thus, by consuming foods with high levels of antioxidants, we are helping protect our cells from damage while maintaining and promoting vitality from within.

HOW ANTIOXIDANTS REDUCE FREE RADICALS

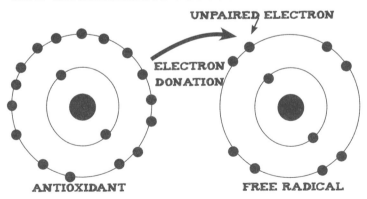

UNPAIRED ELECTRON

ELECTRON DONATION

ANTIOXIDANT

FREE RADICAL

VITAMINS: VITAL COMPONENTS TO OUR HEALTH

Vitamins are a group of compounds essential to the body's performance and function. Classified by what they do rather than their physical structure, vitamins take direct actions on our bodies. For example, vitamin E helps to regenerate cells. Antioxidants, such as vitamins C and A, protect the body from free-radical damage. Vitamins in the B-complex group aid in metabolism, energy production, and nerve functioning.

On the whole, vitamins are unstable and therefore susceptible to degeneration through oxidization, heating (as in cooking), and light. Due to their diverse actions and the body's inability to synthesize on its own, vitamins are truly vital to our health. They are only fully potent as part of the complex cellular structure of plants, and therefore interact differently when isolated. The state a vitamin is in will directly affect the nutritional level it has to offer.

Isabell Shipard, author of *How Can I Grow and Use Sprouts as Living Food?*, has found that sprouted seeds are one of the best and most realistic sources of vitamins, since they can be grown nearly everywhere and by nearly anyone. Through her research, she has discovered that "the vitamin content of some seeds can increase up to twenty times their original weight within days of sprouting. The B vitamin content in mung beans increased compared to dry seeds as follows: B_1 up to 285%, B_2 up to 515% and B_3 256%." In addition, vitamin E and beta-carotene (a precursor to vitamin A) are actively produced during the growth process as the seeds wake up and begin growing into new stages. Even without sprouting, increases in vitamin C and B group vitamins are noted after soaking for eight to twelve hours.

Keep in mind that sprouting isn't limited to raw food. If grains or legumes are to be cooked, it is advantageous to sprout or at least soak the seeds before cooking. While cooking does destroy many heat sensitive vitamins and enzymes, cooking sprouted foods is still a better option than preparing grains from their dry state, for reasons noted above as well as others to be explained in later sections.

> *"Mother Nature is the best physician,*
> *and food is the best medicine."*
> -Dr. Joseph Mercola

ENZYMES: THE FORGOTTEN CAPSTONE IN THE FOOD PYRAMID

Enzymes are large molecules responsible for catalyzing thousands of biochemical reactions in the body, and myriads of functions from blinking to digestion. Enzymes were first named in the late 1870s, stemming from the Greek word for leaven. They are alive, highly active, and specifically designed to carry out certain tasks.

Sprouts are considered living food because they are so rich in enzymes. By consuming highly enzymic foods, such as fresh produce, sprouts, or ferments, we relieve the body of needing to produce its own enzymes. This in turn supports natural cleansing and healing functions, while avoiding the health problems that arise when there is a lack of enzymes such as poor digestion, elimination, toxicity, lethargy, or cellular degeneration.

Digestive enzymes assist in breaking down food, allowing it to dissolve and pass through the intestinal wall into the bloodstream, thus feeding cells. They are co-workers of cells and actually convert food substances into body-building materials. They also help prepare waste to be carried to the kidneys and expelled from of the body. Unlike with vitamins, our body can produce enzymes (in organs like the pancreas), but at an energetic cost and in limited fashion, as the capacity decreases over a lifetime. By reducing the need for the body to produce enzymes, we are reducing the stress load and freeing up energy for regeneration and detoxification.

Ann Wigmore (1909-1994), one of the most significant pioneers in the sprouting movement, spoke of enzymes as worker bees—an integral support of both life and the body. One of her peers Edward Howell played a monumental role in the study of enzymes and their effect on humans, bringing forth the idea that enzymes are promoters of youthfulness and vitality.

People can easily overlook the importance of enzymes in their lives. A lack of enzymes from foods over time results in an overtaxed body that can't properly digest food, leading to low absorption and assimilation of nutrients, and higher levels of free-radical damage, which can ultimately decrease immune function and youthfulness. The solution to overstressing the body's enzyme production is simple: Fill it up with digestive enzymes in the food you eat so they don't need to be manufactured. Eat sprouts!

>>
"All life, whether plant or animal,
requires the presence of enzymes to keep it going."
-Edward Howell, from *Enzyme Nutrition*
<<

MINERALS: THE BONES OF THE EARTH

Minerals are the physical foundation of this Earth—the inorganic substances that form the basis for biological life. Our bodies rely on them to keep our systems balanced and highly functional. Minerals are complex, and serve a wide range of functions (too many to mention here). We can obtain all the necessary minerals (a.k.a. dietary elements) from food. Here are the major ones listed from most to least abundant in our bodies: calcium, phosphorus, potassium, sulfur, sodium, chlorine, and magnesium. We also need these trace, or minor, minerals in much smaller quantities: iron, cobalt, copper, zinc, molybdenum, iodine, bromine, and selenium.

Minerals appear in many forms and are most available to our bodies if they are chelated (bound to a protein). Sprouting greatly increases the chelation of minerals by unlocking them, which allows them to be used by us for our growth and development.

CHLOROPHYLL: NATURE'S HEALING ELIXIR

All sprouts with leaves have the potential to produce chlorophyll if given access to sunlight. This means that you can grow your own nourishing foods, and use the potent abilities of nature to heal and flourish, anywhere you have moderate access to light.

Chlorophyll may be the most miraculous substance on the planet; it plays a crucial role in converting sunlight to usable forms of energy that fuels life on Earth. Commonly seen as the green pigment in leaves, chlorophyll is able to absorb most of the sun's light (green is second to black in light-absorbing qualities). Chemically, chlorophyll is nearly identical to hemoglobin, differing only in that it has a center element of magnesium rather than iron. Its natural cleansing properties have been used by medical doctors for 70 years, both internally and externally to treat wounds, infections, and toxicity.

Due to its similarity to hemoglobin, it acts as an effective blood cleanser by supporting repair and regeneration of red blood cells (which are lacking in anemic people), and allowing for more oxygen to be carried in the bloodstream. Chlorophyll also creates an alkaline environment where toxins are processed and eliminated, and where disease-causing anaerobic bacteria cannot survive. This oxygenating effect has particular merit in regards to toxins and carcinogens stored in the liver (e.g. the aflatoxins in moldy grains and seeds). This highly oxygenated, alkaline environment, therefore, combats infection and boosts overall immunity.

PLANT BLOOD
(CHLOROPHYLL)

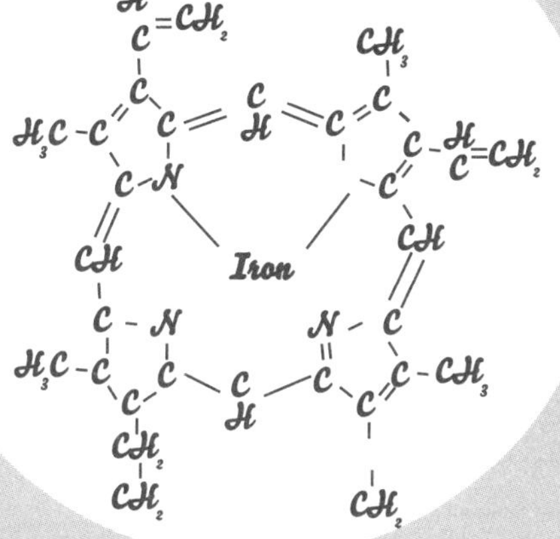

H
$C = CH_2$ CH_3

$H_3C - C$ $C = CH$ $C - C$

$C - N$ $C - H$ $C = CH_2$

CH **Iron** CH

$C - N$ $N - C$

$H_3C - C$ C C $C - CH_3$

CH_2 H

CH_2 CH_2

HUMAN BLOOD
(HEMOGLOBIN)

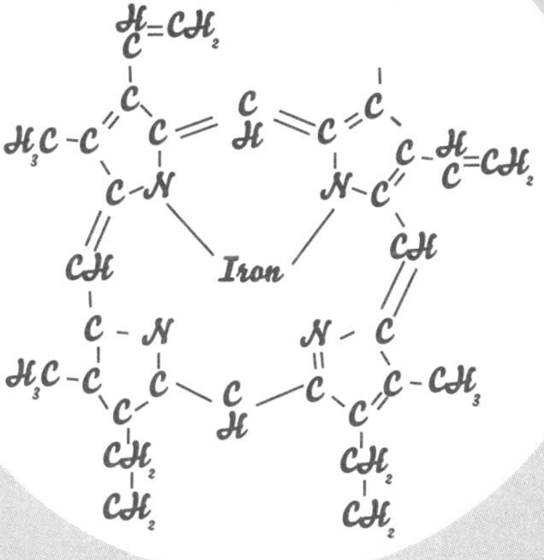

$H = CH_2$

C

$H_3C - C$ $C = C$ $C = C$

$C - N$ $N - C$ $C - H$ $C = CH_2$

CH **Iron** CH

$C - N$ $N - C$

$H_3C - C$ C C C $C - CH_3$

CH_2 H CH_2

CH_2 CH_2

One of chlorophyll's primary actions is to limit the metabolism of harmful compounds that may become carcinogens, thus preventing potential damage to DNA. Chlorophyll has an amazing ability to combine itself with harmful compounds to form large molecules that the small intestines are unable to absorb. A true agent of blood regeneration and youthfulness, chlorophyll revitalizes our bodies from the inside out. Other beneficial effects include improved digestion, decreased inflammation, to a calmer demeanor. Our bodies are meant to consume chlorophyll and green plants are the most accessible source.

PHYTOCHEMICALS: DEFENDERS OF HEALTH

Along with their vitamin- and chlorophyll-production capacities, plants also produce compounds known as phytochemicals. These are produced to protect the plant from pathogens (agents that cause harm or illness), pests, and other natural stresses of the environment. These compounds are often concentrated in the seeds in order to ensure the health of future generations.

Many of these chemicals have immense healing potentials for humans; they protect us against carcinogens and other free-radical damage, and are known sometimes as phytonutrients due to their nourishing qualities. In general, newly germinated plants are more susceptible to predators and stress than mature plants, so they often have higher levels of phytonutrients. These levels are diluted over time as plants take up water and become bulkier.

All vegetables contain beneficial phytonutrients, but broccoli sprouts seem to top the list when it comes to potency. Broccoli has been proven to prevent hypertension, osteoarthritis, heart disease, allergies, ulcers, and diabetes. Broccoli sprouts have also recently been linked to the detoxification of environmental pollutants in the body—awakening and supporting the body's capacity to "take out the trash." In a world where exhaust from cars and all sorts of other air pollutions are nearly unavoidable, you benefit from increasing your body's detoxifying capacity.

Concentrated in the seed and activated during germination, phytochemicals are highly valuable. One such chemical is sulforaphane, which is found in cruciferous vegetables (broccoli, watercress, cabbage, etc.) and alliums (onions, garlic, etc.), as well as their seeds. Sulforaphane is an effective anti-carcinogen because it's capable of inhibiting tumor growth, killing cancer cells, and acting as an antimicrobial agent. In 1997, Dr. Paul Talalay headed a major study through John Hopkins Institute to measure the effectiveness of sulforaphane on known carcinogens. He states: "Three-day-old broccoli sprouts consistently contain twenty to fifty times the amount of chemoprotective compounds found in mature broccoli heads, and may offer a simple, dietary means of chemically reducing cancer risk."

According to alternative-medicine proponent Dr. Joseph Mercola, sulforaphane also supports DNA's methylation by helping cells "remember who they are and where they have been." Imagine photocopying a document. Over time, that document may become smudged, and if you continue to make copies, the smudges manifest and become accentuated. By regulating gene expression and DNA methylation, sulforaphane helps cells make copies of the clean, original source, not of the smudged copy.

Phytoestrogens, such as lignans and isoflavones, are another group of phytochemicals that are found in many fruits and vegetables, and in concentrated levels in soy and leafy legume sprouts (e.g. clover and alfalfa) as well as oilseeds like flax. These chemicals offer significant protection against breast and prostate cancers, as well as aid against moderate symptoms of menopause, osteoporosis, atherosclerosis, and neurodegeneration.

Phytoestrogens act similarly to estrogen in the body, but because they are from an outside source, they are received and processed differently. Their actions are complex and far reaching. (The endocrine system is highly intricate, and too complicated to be able to explain in this book). There is some debate regarding the safety of these compounds, but many studies have proved their protective effects on the body. Many different and naturally occurring chemical compounds work synergistically with each other. This means that phytochemicals do not act alone when offering their preventative and protective effects to our bodies.

The important bit here is to remember that sprouts are self-contained life sources that are full of the fodder to fuel and to protect. I personally don't bother too much with worrying about one particular compound, or contradicting studies that endorse this or condone that. Keep in mind that life is complex and not of human origin; we did not make life, and our understanding of it is limited. Seeds know how to sprout. Our bodies know how to heal. And our minds have the power to confuse. Trust your body and instinct. Eat living plants.

NEUTRALIZING THE ANTINUTRIENTS

Seeds come packed with nutrients that plants use throughout their growth. These nutrients are accompanied by antinutrients such as phytic acid and enzyme inhibitors. Antinutrients can have a harmful effect on our GI tracts, as well as reduce the bioavailability of the nutrients. For example, phytic acid—a compound that is present in all grains, and most seeds and nuts, and is a stable form of phosphorus geared toward nourishing future seedlings—either blocks or binds with zinc, iron, calcium, and magnesium, and make these minerals unavailable to our bodies. Good for plants, but not for us.

Also present in seeds are enzyme inhibitors that prevent premature germination, and that act as deterrents for predators (as is trypsin inhibitor, found in legumes). These qualities make them ideal as herbicides and pesticides. Enzyme inhibitors decrease the activity of enzymes both in food and in our bodies (refer to Enzymes, page 20). Due to their ability to work against metabolic action, these antinutrients should be removed from your food.

Although studies have shown that some antinutrients (i.e. phytic acid) inhibit digestion, reduce bioavailability of nutrients, and are linked to an increased risk in cavities, other "antinutrients," such as protease inhibitors and tannins (found in cacao, tea, grapes, etc.), are said to be potent anti-carcinogens. For our sake, sprouting or simply soaking seeds before consumption allows the natural process of germination to take care of these unhealthy compounds by neutralizing or removing them.

GET SPROUTING!

Hopefully, having read this far, you're ready and excited to try out sprouting for yourself! There is a huge amount of variety and potential as you endeavor forward on your sprouting path. Sprouting is not an isolated act, but a shift towards a more holistic health management strategy and a life that is more connected to the wisdom and rhythms of nature.

The short answer is: You can sprout almost any seed. The options are numerous; most edible seeds in their whole state, as well as cruciferous vegetable seeds, can be sprouted (see Cautions, page 32). The methods of cultivation and preparation vary from seed to seed, but the basics remain the same: Keep seeds moist and in a happy environment, and they will sprout on their own.

SEEDS TO SPROUT

Legumes (eaten as seeds or shoots)

Grains (eaten as seeds or grown as grass for juicing)

Nuts and Seeds (eaten whole, blended, or ground)

Vegetables (eaten young, mostly from the brassica family)

There are a number of ways to make use of sprouts, and each has its advantages. For example, sunflowers and buckwheat can be grown as sprouts in the hulled form, or as microgreens with their hulls. Hulls are fairly indigestible, being composed mostly of protective fiber that encapsulates the seed. They play an important role in safeguarding the seed from environmental damage or premature germination. The various methods of sprouting and the timeframe of growth with each seed also offer diversity in utilizing the full potential of sprouts.

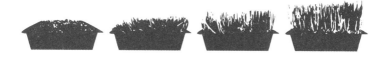

TYPES OF SPROUTS

Sprouts (eaten as tails/radicles begin to emerge)

Microgreens (grown for young shoots and leaves)

Grasses (used for juicing young blades)

METHODS OF SPROUTING

Jars (most accessible option; glass jar with screen top)

Bags (require the most attention to hygiene)

Trays (for microgreens and grasses, multiple medium options)

Commercial sprouters (a variety of models are available)

(Shorter growth times are best in jars, strainer, bags, or commercial sprouters, while longer growth is best supported by trays.)

All sprouts begin with a seed, so start with a high quality seed. Preferably organic seeds, as any harmful agricultural chemical used on the plant or soil tends to accumulate in the seed. Seeds that are too old lose their viability, so make sure you buy seeds grown in the previous growing season when possible.

Use good water. Ideally, fresh spring water is used for sprouting operations, free of heavy metal, chemical, or bacterial contamination. Tap water can be used, but must first be left exposed to air for twenty-four hours, letting all the volatile chlorine molecules evaporate and de-chlorination to occur (chlorine is used to kill the life in water).

As most sprouts will be eaten raw, extra careful attention must be paid to hygiene. Of concern is bacterial contamination such as E. coli.

By washing equipment well and then sterilizing with hot water and/or hydrogen peroxide, sprouts can be grown without threat of contamination. With proper sources and practices, anyone with even the smallest of spaces and access to clean water can produce their own living food all year round at a very economical rate. By following some simple guidelines, success is inevitable.

SUMMARY OF SPROUTING BASICS

Use high quality, organic, responsibly sourced seeds (for cleanliness and consistent germination)

Use clean water (the key to healthy sprouts)

Rinse often (more is better than less)

Maintain good air circulation (stagnant air is attractive to molds and bacteria)

USING SPROUTS

Sprouts are not an addition to food, they are food; as such, there are infinite ways to use them to create luscious, and healthy dishes that promote vitality. Sprouting is not limited to raw foods, nor should the idea of sprouting be limited to what is popular or most well known. Once the basics are understood, you may develop your own tastes, style and approach to incorporating sprouting into everyday life.

The more delicate greens are best left uncooked, eaten whole, blended or juiced. The enzymic activity is particularly sensitive on produce like microgreens, so treat them as living beings. Leaves combine well with any food, so finding ways to eat microgreens in salads, soups, and sandwiches isn't difficult.

The other products may require some stretching to fit into your food repertoire, but once introduced they are simple enough to include in daily food preparation. Sprouted crackers, desserts and mylks can easily be substituted for conventional options. Grains can be prepared as usual, simply use pre-sprouted grains when preparing grain dishes. Sprouting becomes a part of your lifestyle and soon becomes second nature, allowing for creativity to flow through.

All sprouts have their unique needs, flavors and uses, so the possibilities for combinations are limitless. Legumes, like lentils, can be a fresh crunch to salads and or a cooling touch to hot foods, like soups and stews. Some legumes are particularly difficult to digest (like soy or kidney beans) and will still need to be broken down by cooking or fermentation. These and other cooked legumes are always best to sprout first and then prepare as normal.

CAUTIONS: WHAT TO BE AWARE OF

Recent media attention draws concern to the health issues of sprouting. Cases of E. coli have been linked to sprout consumption, but this is more an issue of hygiene and contaminated water than sprouting itself. For the home sprouter, it is easily avoided by observing proper hygiene. According to the Sproutman, Steve Meyerowitz, "In a given year, getting hit by lightning (1.29 people per million) is more likely than contracting E. Coli (1.1 people per million) from meat, poultry, shellfish, milk, eggs, and produce combined." Vegetarian foods propose an even lower risk of contamination.

Alfalfa has also received negative attention due to the presence of the toxin canavanine. Realistically, it is said to occur in such a low concentration that it is not of significant concern, yet some critics still advise against its consumption at all. The FDA warns against consuming alfalfa for the young, the elderly, pregnant or lactating mothers and those with compromised immunity, especially those with dormant systemic lupus. However, the damaging effects are noted upon consuming 14,000 milligrams of canavanine. Considering that a healthy serving of alfalfa may contain two or three milligrams, it would take 7,000 servings of alfalfa sprouts within a twenty-four period to get enough of the toxin to harm your body. Taking this into account, you may draw your own conclusions.

Some beans contain reasonable amounts of toxins (enough to avoid raw consumption of them), such as those from the phaseolus genus like kidney beans and black beans. These are best eaten well-soaked, rinsed and thoroughly cooked with an herbal or mineral neutralizing agent, such as asafoetida, baking soda, vinegar, epizote, sea weed, etc. These help neutralize possibly harmful compounds, as well as assist in breaking down the complex starches that may cause gas and bloating. The safest and most digestible legumes are lentils (lens genus), adzuki and mung beans (vigna genus). Some legumes are simply better tolerated lightly cooked, as the complex starches are further broken down by cooking. Some people prefer not to eat raw chickpeas, but instead sprout them before cooking.

Lastly, some peas have received negative press due to their correlation with various outbreaks of lathyrism, a condition that paralyses the lower extremities. The main cause of lathyrism globally is the consumption of large amounts of Lathyrism Sativus, commonly known as grass pea, blue sweet pea, chickling vetch or Indian pea. Grass pea is a drought tolerant food that can be consumed safely if properly leached of toxins. Unfortunately, when drought conditions arise this is one readily available food, and improper preparation (omitting the boiling and leaching process to conserve water) leads to outbreaks as seen in China (1972–1974), Ethiopia (1976), Afghanistan (1998), Nepal (1998) and Ethiopia (1997–1999). In other instances, ornamental garden plants that have been mistakenly sold as chickpeas contain toxins that cause lathyrism.

HYDROPONIC SPROUTING

The hydroponic method, using jars or sprouting bags, is the simplest place to start with sprouting. All you need is water, easily obtainable equipment, some patience, and a little bit of information. It's the gateway to the sprouting world, and you may have all the materials in your kitchen already. Best results will be had in temperatures ranging from 60°F to 80°F / 15°C to 26°C.

Each seed has its own characteristics and timing. Some seeds should be allowed to leaf out and produce chlorophyll, while others can be eaten as radicles emerge. Nuts will only swell, not growing tails at all. Refer to the sprout chart on pages 118–119.

SOME SEEDS TO START WITH

SUNFLOWERS

A classic seed grown in North America, sunflowers are economical and can be eaten creamy or crunchy. They're high in protein, fat, vitamin E, and minerals. Great as an added crunch to cereals and salads, blended as a base for non-dairy mylks, sauces and dressings, or added to bread and crackers.

LENTILS

A great choice for beginners because lentils will sprout within a day, creating juicy and succulent munchies. (Note that split lentils will not sprout.) A good source of protein and containing thirty times more vitamin C when sprouted, lentils can be eaten out of hand, in salads, or ground into crackers and breads.

BROCCOLI

Densely packed with vitamins and protective phytochemicals with plenty of room to spare for flavor, broccoli is the most concentrated source of several cancer combating ingredients. A great addition to salads, soups, sandwiches, and just about anything you put in your mouth.

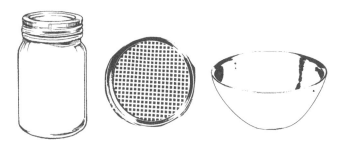

JAR METHOD

MATERIALS

- 1 Quart / 1 L wide mouth mason jars
- Stainless steel or non-resonated nylon screen (NOT galvanized steel)
- Bowl or container to rest jars in
- Seeds for sprouting (organic is preferred)

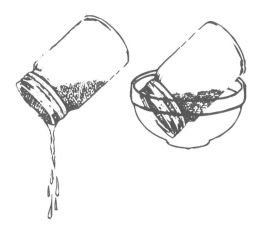

PROCESS

Step 1: Soak

Place 2–4 tablespoons of small seeds or ½ cup of legumes, large seeds, or grains per 1 L / quart jar. Place seeds in jar, and then fill up two to three times as much as the seeds with water. Replace solid lid with screen and secure with screw top or elastic. Soak in a dark place for 4 to 6 hours with small seeds, 4 to 8 hours with sunflower and pumpkin, and 12 or more hours with larger legumes and grains (see chart in Appendix).

Step 2: Rinse

Pour out water, refill, wash, and drain until water runs off clear.

Step 3: Drain

Leave jar to drain fully at a 45° angle, or less if there is any remaining water that needs to be drained. Seeds should be moist but not soaking to allow airflow and discourage bacterial growth.

Step 4: Rinse

Repeat this rinse and drain cycle (steps three and four) for 8 to 12 hours, or more frequently if very hot. Legumes and grains reach their nutrient potential when the tail is at least as long as the seed.

Step 5: Greening

For small leafy greens (brassicas, clovers, etc.), this is a crucial step for chlorophyll production. After 3 or 4 days of growth, simply expose the sprouts to indirect sunlight, and they will produce their own chlorophyll!

Step 6: Dehull

For small leafy greens, this step extends shelf life dramatically, as hulls hold excess water that can lead to spoilage. Place seeds in a large bowl and fill with cool water. Lightly agitate the seeds to allow the indigestible hulls to float to the surface. Skim off and compost hulls. Return to jar for final rinse, or dry in salad spinner. Most sprouts will keep fresh for 7 to 10 days if covered, but are best eaten fresh.

Step 7: Harvest

For legumes, large seeds, and grains, skip Steps 5 and 6 and place in a covered container in the fridge until eaten.

NOTES

- For larger seeds, the same instructions can be followed using a colander or sieve in place of glass jar.

- Brassica seeds will grow fuzzy root hairs after two days. This is not mold; just make sure to rinse thoroughly to avoid clumping.

- Sunflower seeds should not be allowed to grow longer than a day unless planted for greens, because mold can easily develop on the seeds.

- Experiment with different combinations of sprouts in the same jar if the maturation times are similar for flavor and texture. This also aids in avoiding clumping and allows better air circulation.

- Sprouting screen lids can be purchased (see Resources, page 124), or you can make your own by cutting food-safe plastic labeled #2 (HPDE) or #5 (PP) to fit over the wide mouth jar and drilling small drainage holes.

VARIATION

Use a tube instead of a jar to allow an increase of air circulation and drainage. The tube can be made of any dense plastic considered safe for plumbing uses. For safety reasons, avoid any flexible tubes that may contain phthalates, a dangerous and toxic substance present in many flexible plastics. The sizing of the tube can be 3 in to 4 in (7.5 cm to 10 cm) wide and any length that is convenient for your operation. Plumbing pipes, such as PVC tubing, will do and can be fitted with caps on one end, serving to hold water for the initial soak. The other end can be fitted with a screen similar to the jar method. Once the seeds are done soaking, invert the tube, remove the cap, and continue as directed above.

SPROUTING BAGS

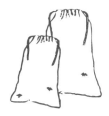

The most compact and simple kinds of sprouter, these loosely woven drawstring bags are usually about 6 in (15 cm) wide and 9 in (22 cm) tall, and made from linen, bamboo, cotton, hemp, and non-resonated nylon. Choose a fabric that is durable, holds water, and can be washed frequently to avoid bacteria accumulation. Bamboo is a good choice because it is a sustainable fiber and has anti-fungal properties. Sprout bags are ideal for traveling or low maintenance operations.

To grow sprouts in a bag, follow the same steps as with the jar method: Simply place a bag in a bowl to soak and rinse, and then hang up to drain. Bags work best for grains and legumes, although leafy greens are possible with more attention to hygiene.

WHAT TO GROW HYDROPONICALLY

MUNG AND ADZUKI BEANS

Mung beans are the most commonly grown bean sprouts. To achieve the plump and blanched sprouts, the method varies slightly from the jar method. These delights can be grown into long, crisp and full sprouts in 3 to 5 days. Best results are achieved if kept in low-lit areas (production of chlorophyll stimulates cellulose development, making stalks tough) and under pressure (to strengthen stalks).

MATERIALS

- Colander or basket with drainage
- Plate, or similar object, that fits inside a colander or basket
- Weight (clean brick, rock, jar of water, etc.)

PROCESS

Step 1: Sprout

Sprout as previously instructed for 3 days, rinsing with cold water three times daily.

Step 2: Apply Weight

On the third day of sprouting, cover seeds with a container, plate or a second pot and then apply weight. Another jar filled with water, a clean masonry brick or any heavy object will do. Remove weight to rinse.

Step 3: Dehull

Once they have reached desired length (1 in to 3 in / 1.5 cm to 4.5 cm), place in a large bowl filled with cold water to remove the hulls. This will improve taste and storage time. Lightly agitate to allow hulls to rise to the top as sprouts settle and separate from their hulls. Skim off hulls and compost. Drain sprouts fully and store in a sealed container in the fridge.

NUTS AND SEEDS

Most nuts and seeds are difficult to digest if not sprouted. In their dried forms, they contain high levels of enzyme inhibitors, which force the body to produce hydrochloric acid and bile needed to break down these complex foods. Some notable exceptions are flax and chia, which can be easily assimilated when ground (chia can actually be eaten whole). Nuts and seeds generally do not sprout tails (sunflowers will, but should not be allowed to grow this long unless intended for microgreens). Fortunately, they do go through the necessary alchemy needed to become easily digestible and therefore useful to the body. Some sources suggest soaking nuts in brine (a salt-water solution) as the Aztecs did. The nuts can then be dried and stored for later use.

Step 1: Soak

For 1 C / 250 ml raw nuts, use 1 ½ tsp / 7.5 ml salt, and enough water to cover generously. Soak according to chart on pages 118–119.

Step 2: Drain

You have the option here to leave the nuts slightly salty or to rinse the salt off.

Step 3: Dry

Spread the nuts in a single layer on a baking sheet. Dry them on a warm setting 160°F / 70°C for 12 to 24 hours until crispy. Store in an airtight container.

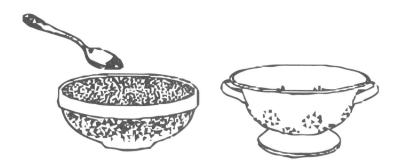

RECIPES

SAUCES & DIPS

LENTIL HUMMUS

A spinoff of the classical hummus. Because of the unpleasant "legumey" taste of raw beans, it is best to pulse in a food processor and rinse off the starch. or else steam the beans for 5 to 10 minutes.

INGREDIENTS

- 2 C / 500 ml sprouted lentils (or chickpeas)
- 1 ¼ / 300 ml quartered tomatoes
- 1 C / 250 ml thick mylk (see Recipes, page 94)
- ¼ C / 60 ml tahini (raw or roasted)
- 3 Tbsp / 45 ml olive oil
- 2 Tbsp / 60 ml lemon juice
- 1 ½ to 2 cloves of garlic
- 1 tsp / 5 ml white pepper
- 1 tsp / 5 ml salt
- 1 tsp / 5 ml cumin powder

PROCESS
Step 1: Puree
Place lentils and mylk in food processor, followed by remaining ingredients (this may have to be done in two batches). Puree until smooth.

Step 2: Serve

Hummus is a great addition to anything! Spread on crackers or breads, or use as a dip for raw veggies. If serving as a dip, garnish with a drizzling of olive oil and a sprinkling of cumin.

....

VEGAN RAITA

An Indian creamy and cooling sauce usually made from yogurt. Raita is a great compliment to hot and spicy dishes, and can also be eaten with lentil crackers (see recipe, page 89) or as a sauce for mixed sprouts.

INGREDIENTS

- 1 ¼ C / 560 ml almonds

- ¾ C water

- 2 Tbsp / 30 ml apple cider vinegar

- 1 large cucumber, peeled

- ¼ C / 60 ml mint, finely chopped

- ¼ C / 60 ml cilantro or fennel, finely chopped

- 1 tsp / 5 ml ground cumin

- ½ tsp / 2.5 ml salt

PROCESS

Thoroughly blend all ingredients until lusciously smooth.

GREEN DIP

INGREDIENTS

- 2 C / 500 ml sprouted peas
- ½ C / 125 ml sprouted sunflower seeds
- ½ C / 125 ml spinach or kale, finely chopped
- 2 Tbsp / 30 ml extra virgin olive oil
- 1 Tbsp / 15 ml tamari or nama shoyu
- 1 medium onion
- 1 to 3 garlic cloves
- 1 Tbsp / 15 ml dried dill

PROCESS

Step 1: Puree

Place everything in food processor and puree until smooth.

Step 2: Serve

Spread on crackers or breads, or use as a dip for raw veggies.

ENTREES

SPROUTED BEAN RICE BOWL

*This bowl is a simple, grounding, and nourishing stand-alone food. On
a bed of brown rice balanced with sprouts and topped with gomashio (a
Japanese seasoning, commonly identified as sea salt), this dish adheres to
the Macrobiotic style of eating. Gomashio can be made in large batches and
used as table condiment, replacing salt.
Recipe adapted from sproutpeople.com*

INGREDIENTS

- 1 C / 250 ml bean, pea, or lentil sprouts

- ½ C / 125 ml brown rice (short grain is my favorite)

- ½ C / 125 ml vegetable of choice (optional)

- ¼ C / 60 ml raw sesame seeds, soaked and well drained

- +/- ½ Tbsp / 7.5 ml salt

PROCESS

Step 1: Cook rice

Rinse rice well, and then bring 1 C / 250 ml water to a boil. Reduce heat
and simmer for 45 minutes.

Step 2: Make gomashio

Heat skillet (ideally cast iron) over medium heat for 1 to 2 minutes. Add
sesame seeds, and stir constantly to avoid burning. Once they pop and turn
golden brown (1 to 2 minutes), remove them from skillet. Lightly toast
the salt until fragrant. This will "cool" the salt, or bring more yin energy
according to the Traditional Chinese Medicine or Macrobiotic perspective.
If you're lucky enough to have a suribachi, use it! If not, a mortar and

pestle, or food processor, will work. Grind until you're satisfied, or don't grind at all—it's about preference. Ratio of sesame to salt may vary from 5:1 to 15:1, so find what suits you best. This recipe is about 8:1.

Step 3: Finalize

During the last 5 minutes or so of cooking, add veggies (if using) and steam lightly. You may also choose to lightly steam the sprouts for 2 minutes, but that's a personal choice; they're good either way. Now for the best part—eating it. Serve sprouted-bean rice bowl with gomashio.

LENTIL QUINOA TABOULI

INGREDIENTS

- 2 C / 500 ml sprouted lentils (French are my favorite)
- 2 C / 500 ml cooked quinoa or millet
- ¼ C / 60 ml sprouted sunflower seeds
- 1 cucumber, peeled and cubed
- 2 scallions, sliced thinly
- 2 medium tomatoes, cubed
- 1 C / 250 ml chopped parsley
- 2 cloves of garlic
- 4 Tbsp / 60 ml olive oil
- 4 Tbsp / 60 ml apple cider vinegar or lemon
- 2 tsp / 10 ml dried oregano or thyme
- 1 tsp / 5 ml salt
- 1 tsp / 5 ml black pepper

PROCESS

Chop tomatoes and cucumbers into ½ in / 1.75 cm cubes. Dice garlic, scallions, and parsley. Mix all ingredients thoroughly and set to marinate a few hours.

DAHL

This classic Indian soup staple takes the addition of legume sprouts
wonderfully. Dahl is usually made from lentils, but can also be made from
mung or adzuki beans. This soft and comforting food has been a standby
for generations.

INGREDIENTS

- 4 C / 1 L sprouted lentils, adzuki, or mung beans
- 1 C / 250 ml water or vegetable stock
- 1 onion, finely diced
- 2 medium tomatoes, diced (optional)
- 4 cloves garlic, finely diced or crushed
- 2 Tbsp / 30 ml coconut, sunflower or olive oil
- 1 Tbsp / 15 ml fresh ginger, shredded
- 1 tsp / 5 ml cumin
- 1 tsp / 5 ml coriander
- 1 tsp / 5 ml turmeric
- Salt to taste

PREPARATION

Step 1: Cook seasonings

In a saucepan or pot, add oil and spices, and heat on medium-high heat until spices become fragrant (3 to 5 minutes). Add ginger and onions and cook until translucent.

Step 2: Cook dahl

Add lentil sprouts, water/stock, and tomatoes (if using). Cook another 5 to 10 minutes until lentils become tender, or cook less if crunchiness is desired. Goes great with flatbread, crackers or rice.

BARLEY AND VEGETABLE SOUP

A comforting winter standby, able to nourish and warm the body and soul.
An excellent example of using sprouts in a soup recipe.

INGREDIENTS

- 6 C / 1 ½ L water, stock, or broth
- 2 C / 500 ml sprouted barley
- 1 C white wine
- 4 medium carrots, diced into 1-in (2.5-cm) cubes
- 3 medium onions, diced into 1-in (2.5-cm) cubes
- 2 medium parsnips, diced into 1-in (2.5-cm) cubes
- ¼ C / 60 ml olive oil
- 2 Tbsp / 30 ml rosemary
- 2 Tbsp / 30 ml oregano or marjoram
- 1 Tbsp / 15 ml caraway seeds (optional)
- 2 tsp / 10 ml ground black pepper
- 1 tsp / 5 ml kelp powder
- Salt to taste

PREPARATION

Step 1: Saute onion

In a soup pot on low heat, saute onion, pepper, and caraway seed with oil until onions become translucent.

Step 2: Add vegetables

Add carrots and parsnips to pot, and then cook for 5 minutes.

Step 3: Add seasoning
Add wine, herbs, and salt to mixture. Cook until liquid is reduced by half.

Step 4: Cook barley
Add water, stock or broth, and barley. Cook until barley reaches desired tenderness, about 30 to 45 minutes.

....

SALADS

WALDORF SALAD

INGREDIENTS

- 2 C / 500 ml sprouted buckwheat

- 2 tart apples, cubed

- 1 C / 250 ml soaked raisins (in ½ C / 125 ml water)

- 1 C walnuts, soaked and rinsed

- 1 C / 250 ml fresh parsley, chopped

- 3 Tbsp / 45 ml apple cider vinegar

- 2 Tbsp / 30 ml extra-virgin olive oil

- 2 Tbsp / 30 ml ground flax seed

- ½ tsp / 2.5 ml salt

- ½ tsp / 2.5 ml ground black pepper

- ½ tsp / 2.5 ml ground nutmeg

- ½ tsp / 2.5 ml ground cinnamon

PROCESS

Combine buckwheat, apples, and walnuts in a large bowl. Drain raisins and add to bowl. Combine soak water with all wet ingredients. Mix in spices and pour over salad. Toss well and serve.

....

MUNG BEAN CILANTRO SALAD

A cooling, refreshing, and detoxifying salad.

INGREDIENTS

- 2 C / 500 ml mung bean sprouts
- 1 handful leafy sprouts (radish, broccoli, clover)
- 1 cucumber, cubed
- 1 C / 250 ml cilantro, chopped
- 1 Tbsp / 15 ml garlic (2 medium cloves), minced
- 1 Tbsp / 15 ml fresh ginger, grated
- ¼ C / 60 ml lemon juice
- 2 Tbsp / 30 ml tamari or nama shoyu

PROCESS

Chop cucumbers into ½-in / 1.75-cm cubes. Finely chop cilantro and mix all ingredients thoroughly. Set aside to marinate a few hours. If you don't have time, that's fine—it's still tasty.

SNACKS

SEASONED SPROUTS

This mixture is great on its own, as a topping for entrees and stir-fries, or as a rice add-in. Adapted from "Spicy San Francisco Sprout Snack" from sproutpeople.org

INGREDIENTS

- 4 C / 1 L sprouted legumes (beans, lentils, or peas—combined or solo*)
- 2 C soaked almonds**
- 1 Tbsp / 15 ml garlic powder
- 1 Tbsp / 15 ml onion powder
- 1 Tbsp / 15 ml chili powder (chipotle, if possible)
- 1 Tbsp / 15 ml thyme (finely ground)
- 1 Tbsp / 15 ml salt
- 1 Tbsp / 15 ml pepper
- 1 Tbsp / 15 ml whole cane sugar (optional)
- 1 Tbsp / 15 ml cayenne pepper
- 1 ½–3 tsp / 7.5–15 m ml hot sauce
- 2–3 tsp / 10–15 ml olive oil

*Approximately 2 C / 500 ml dry
** Approximately 1 ¼ C / 185 ml dry

PREPARATION
Step 1: Sprout
Soak legumes and sprout for 24 hours. Soak almonds.

Step 2: Mix

Mix all ingredients together by sprinkling powders over sprout mixture. Toss to mix evenly.

....

TERYAKI ALMONDS

A wonderfully gourmet preparation of almonds, sure to deliver full flavor and a satisfying crunch. These seasoned nuts make a stunning final touch to stir-fries, salads, soups, or baked vegetables.

INGREDIENTS

- 2 ½ C / 600 ml almonds
- ¼ C / 60 ml palm sugar
- ¼ C / 60 ml nutritional yeast
- 2 Tbsp / 30 ml tamari or nama shoyu
- 2 Tbsp / 30 ml chia seeds
- 1 Tbsp / 15 ml miso
- 2–4 garlic cloves (depending on size, potency, and preference)
- 1 ½ tsp / 7.5 ml fresh ginger, minced
- 1 tsp / 5ml smoked paprika

PROCESS

Step 1: Soak

Cover seeds with water and soak overnight.

Step 2: Drain

Drain, rinse, and allow to air.

Step 3: Season

Finely chop, dice, or shred the garlic. Mix all ingredients thoroughly.

Step 4: Dry

Spread in thick clusters on dehydrator tray and dehydrate them for 12 to 24 hours, or use an oven at 160°F / 70°C for 12 to 24 hours until crispy. They should dry as little clusters as the chia absorbs some of the moisture and binds all the ingredients together. Store in an airtight container.

SPROUT BARK

This bark is far more economical than store-bought options, and is a fantastic travel and snack food: crunchy, crispy, and full of life! Eat mounded high with greens, use as a dip delivery system, or add to soups as a balancing element. Stored in an airtight container, these will last several months, possibly longer.

INGREDIENTS

- 2 C / 500 ml lentils

- 1 C / 250 ml sunflower seeds

- 1 C / 250 ml pumpkin seeds

- ½ C / 125 ml nutritional yeast

- ¼ C / 60 ml ground flax

- 2 Tbsp / 30 ml apple cider vinegar

- 2 Tbsp / 30 ml coconut or olive oil

- 2 Tbsp / 30 ml water

- 1 Tbsp / 15 ml dried thyme

- 1 Tbsp / 15 ml tamari or nama shoyu

- 2 tsp / 10 ml cumin

- 1 tsp / 5 ml black pepper, freshly ground

- A handful of fresh herbs, chopped (optional)

PROCESS
Step 1: Sprout
Soak lentils overnight and sprout as usual for 24 hours until tails appear. On the second day when almost ready to eat, soak sunflower seeds for 4 to 8 hours. Rinse and drain.

Step 2: Grind

In batches, grind sunflower seeds and lentils as finely as possible in a food processor, adding liquids and spices along with them. Withhold the flax until the end, as it binds the mixture.

Step 3: Dry

Spread mixture ¼ in / 0.75 cm thick onto nonstick dehydrator sheets (teflex, silicon, or parchment paper) and place onto top of dehydrator trays or baking sheets. Dehydrate at 100°F / 37°C for 12 to 16 hours until crispy. If using an oven, use warming tray or leave the light on with the door slightly ajar.

AZTEC PEPITAS

The freshest and most delicious pumpkin seeds, or pepitas, are richly forest green in color. Many stores carry old Chinese seeds, which work but are not ideal. This recipe makes for a superbly delicious item to stock in your pantry, use in dishes, add to trail mixes or cereals, or enjoy solo.

INGREDIENTS

- 1 C / 250 ml raw pumpkin seeds
- 3 Tbsp to 4 Tbsp / 45 ml to 60 ml nutritional yeast
- 2 tsp salt (exotic volcanic or smoked salts truly bring flavor to the next level)
- 1 tsp to 2 tsp /5 ml to 10 ml chili powder, chipotle, cayenne, paprika

PROCESS

Step 1: Soak
Cover seeds with water and mix in salt. Soak 6 hours.

Step 2: Drain
Drain as usual, but do not rinse.

Step 3: Season
Mix the yeast and chili thoroughly. The potency of the spice depends on the type and quantity of chili used. Chili flakes will work, but do not give an even distribution of heat. I find chipotle to be the most fantastically paired chili with Hawaiian red volcanic salt.

Step 4: Dry
Dry the pepitas in the sun (if possible), dehydrate them for 12 to 24 hours, or use an oven at 160°F / 70°C for 12 to 24 hours until crispy. Store in an airtight container once crispy, and don't eat them all at once.

FANCY FRUIT LEATHER

Chewy and substantial, this is certainly no ordinary fruit leather.

INGREDIENTS

- 1 C / 125 ml buckwheat
- 1 C / 125 ml cashews
- ½ C / 125 ml dates, pitted and roughly chopped
- ½ C / 125 ml figs, destemmed and roughly chopped
- ½ C / 125 ml unsulfured apricots roughly chopped
- ½ C / 125 ml sunflower oil
- $^1/_{10}$ tsp / 0.5 ml fine pink himalayan salt
- 2 tsp / 10 ml pure vanilla extract
- 1 tsp / 5 ml ground cardamom (optional)

PROCESS

Step 1: Sprout

Sprout buckwheat 1 to 2 days ahead of time. Soak cashews for 3 to 4 hours, and then rinse.

Step 2: Grind

Grind all ingredients in food processor until the dough sticks to itself.

Step 3: Dry

Spread in an even ¼-in / 0.6-cm layer on dehydrator sheet or wax paper. Dry until removes easily from sheet and flip. Ready when slightly firm but still pliable.

CHOCOLATE LOVE PIES

Heavenly delicious, highly nutritious, and simply divine. A superb way to treat yourself—a rich and creamy filling resting upon a soft and yielding crust. Makes 24 mini pies.

INGREDIENTS FOR CRUST

- ½ C / 125 ml walnuts or pecans
- ½ C / 125 ml hazelnuts or almonds
- 4 medjool dates
- 2 Tbsp / 30 ml coconut, shredded
- 1 Tbsp / 15 ml cacao powder
- 1 tsp / 5 ml vanilla extract
- A pinch of mixed spice (cinnamon, allspice, nutmeg, etc.) and salt

PROCESS

Step 1: Soak

Soak nuts 8 to 12 hours and rinse, then pat dry with a towel.

Step 2: Grind

Place all ingredients except cacao in a food processor and combine until breadcrumb-like. Add the cacao and pulse till mixed thoroughly. The mix should stick together. If not, pulse more. Press into the base of a 24-piece mini muffin pan. Place in fridge while you make the filling.

INGREDIENTS FOR FILLING

- 2 C / 500 ml raw cashews

- ½ C / 125 ml water

- ½ C / 125 ml maple syrup, or sweetener of your choice

- 2 tsp / 10 ml vanilla extract

- ¼ C / 60 ml raw cacao powder

- ½ C / 125 ml coconut oil (warmed till liquid)

- A pinch of salt

PROCESS
Step 1: Blend

Add all ingredients except the liquid coconut oil and cacao in a blender. Blend ingredients until creamy, then add coconut oil and cacao. Blend again until well combined.

Step 2: Mold

Pour mixture into muffin pans and freeze for about 3 hours. Before serving, place in fridge for 30 minutes and decorate with your favorite topping—soaked nuts, cacao nibs, dehydrated buckwheat, berries, or a chocolate sauce. Mmmmmmm.

RAW CARROT CAKE

INGREDIENTS FOR CAKE

- 3 C / 750 ml carrots, roughly chopped
- 1 C / 250 ml walnuts or pecans*
- 1 C / 250 ml coconut, shredded or flaked
- 1 C / 250 ml pumpkin seeds
- 2 C / 500 ml pitted prunes
- 2 Tbsp / 30 ml ground flax
- 2 Tbsp / 30 ml water
- 3 tsp / 15 ml ground cinnamon
- 2 tsp / 10 ml vanilla extract
- ½ tsp / 2.5 ml ground ginger
- ¼ tsp / 1.25 ml allspice
- ¼ tsp / 1.25 ml ground cardamom

*You may want to reserve a few to top the cake.

PROCESS

Place all ingredients in a food processor and grind, stopping occasionally to scrape the sides and mix in edges. Once sufficiently ground (personal preference), place in 12-in x 8 ½-in / 30-cm x 20-cm, or similarly sized, baking dish lined with parchment paper.

INGREDIENTS FOR ICING

- 2 C / 500 ml cashews

- 1 Tbsp / 15 ml coconut oil

- 2 Tbsp / 30 ml maple, agave syrup, or honey

- 2 medjool dates

- 2 tsp / 10 ml vanilla extract

PROCESS

Soak cashews for 3 to 4 hours. Drain and rinse. Blend all ingredients thoroughly. Spread over cake or cupcakes, and store in refrigerator. Once cooled, cut and remove from dish to serve.

ALMOND BUCKWHEAT BALLS

Little balls chock full of awesomeness. Great to make, and to take on hikes and active adventures. Makes 16 to 20.

INGREDIENTS

- ½ C / 125 ml almonds
- ½ C / 125 ml buckwheat
- 1 C / 250 ml medjool dates, pitted (about 14)
- ½ C / 125 ml unsweetened shredded coconut
- ¼ C / 60 ml raisins or goji berries
- ¼ C / 60 ml dried unsulfured apricots
- 2 tsp / 10 ml pure vanilla extract
- 1 tsp / 5 ml cinnamon
- ½ tsp / 2.5 ml cardamom
- A pinch of salt

PROCESS

Step 1: Sprout

Sprout buckwheat 1 to 2 days ahead of time. Soak almonds 12 hours before beginning. Drain and rinse.

Step 2: Grind

Grind all ingredients in food processor until the dough sticks to itself.

Step 3: Form

With wet hands (to avoid sticking), pinch off golf-ball-size pieces and use your palms to roll them into balls. Coat the outside with shredded coconut for nice finishing touch.

SPROUTED BUCKWHEAT CUPCAKES

*These sweet and wholesome goodies are a fantastic snack that satisfies
hunger and the occasional sweet tooth. Simple to make, and will keep in
fridge for at least a week. Makes 12.*

INGREDIENTS

- 1 C / 250 ml buckwheat
- ½ C / 125 ml sunflower seeds
- 2 Tbsp / 30 ml ground flax seeds
- 1 Tbsp / 15 ml coconut oil, warmed
- 2 C / 500 ml unsweetened coconut, shredded
- 1 apple, grated
- 6 medjool dates, soaked and pitted
- ½ tsp / 2.5 ml cinnamon
- ¼ tsp / 1.25 ml vanilla extract

PROCESS

Step 1: Sprout

Sprout buckwheat 1 ½ to 2 days. Soak sunflower seeds 4 to 8 hours, rinse
and drain thoroughly. Both should be fairly dry to the touch.

Step 2: Grind and mold

In a food processor, combine all of the ingredients and grind until a sticky
dough develops. Spoon dough into a muffin pan with 12 spaces. Refrigerate
several hours before enjoying. If you want to ice cupcakes with creamy
frosting, play around with honey, coconut oil, almond butter, dates, and the
like until you find something that works for you.

INDOOR GREENS

This option allows for the growing of seeds past the germination phase and into the early growth phase of the plant. The young plants are harvested either as grass (as in wheat grass), microgreens (broccoli, clover, etc.), or shoots (sunflower, pea, etc.). The seeds are allowed to release their plumule, as the radicle takes root. Tray sprouting requires only slightly more equipment than methods using bags or jars such as a tray to hold medium, a cover, and the medium itself. Sprouting remains the same: Keep seeds moist, maintain good air circulation, and expose to light.

Greens can be grown all year round, in any space with access to water and indirect light. Greens reach maturity in 5 to 12 days (given adequate heat) and provide a great source of salad or juice, right from your own kitchen. They're also ideal for green soups and adding to wraps or sandwiches. Best of all, they don't need to be shipped across the continent in trucks.

Trays can be standard 10-in x 20-in / 25-cm x 50-cm greenhouse trays, cafeteria trays or reused plastic containers. Some commercial sprouters are sold as solid strainer trays and don't require a medium. The seeds are planted on top of the medium and grow until they are cut at the base of the stem to harvest.

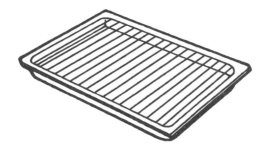

GROWING MICROGREENS

MATERIALS

- Unhulled or whole seeds
- Plastic trays both with and without drainage (most common size is 10 in x 20 in / 25 cm x 50 cm)
- Growing medium (topsoil, coir, vermiculite, etc.)
- Cover for trays (other trays, cloth, etc.)

OR

- Commercial tray-type sprouter

Step 1: Soak

Seeds do best when soaked before planted. The larger the seed, the longer the soak time. Large seeds like peas, sunflowers, and grains are best soaked 8 to 12 hours, while smaller seeds only 4 to 6 hours. Brassicas can drown if soaked too long, and some sources recommend as little as 2 hours for soaking.

Step 2: Prepare Medium

Spread medium ½ in to 1 ½ in / 0.75 cm to 3.25 cm thick evenly along the tray (or lay blanket). Water enough to moisten growing medium fully without making it swampy. I find it best to use a tray with drainage holes to hold the medium and seeds, set into a solid tray to catch excess water.

Step 3: Plant

Drain seeds and spread densely and evenly over growing medium, so that they are touching but not overlapping and competing. Touch seeds lightly to ensure even surface contact. Cover with another tray or plastic to hold in moisture, provide mild weight, and keep light out while sprouting begins. This allows more consistent germination. A weighted cover will force roots to press into the medium more thoroughly. Several trays stacked one upon another work well.

Step 4: Uncover

Periodically check to ensure moisture is adequate. The medium should remain moist, so water as needed. Uncover the tray once the sprouts begin to push up on the cover (usually after 3 days or so) and expose it to indirect light—i.e. sunlight or an artificial-light source. The more light available, the fuller and quicker the growth will be.

Step 5: Water

The amount of water needed depends on heat, growing medium, and airflow. Make sure that the medium stays constantly moist, but not soggy. The greens will suffer if moisture-level of the medium isn't correct. Water using a mister and light with an overhead device (or light from the bottom if using the two-tray system). The earlier stages are done by misting. Later stages require watering from the bottom. This keeps out excess moisture from the leaves, and reduces risk of mold or bacterial growth.

Step 6: Harvest

Keep the medium moist until the green leaves have fully expanded and completely shed their hulls. Grasses are ready when they have reached 4 in to 6 in / 10 cm to 13 cm in height, and greens at 2 in to 4 in / 5 cm to 10 cm. Handle grasses or greens carefully, and cut with a sharp knife or scissors just above the soil line. Some trays can be harvested again as seeds re-grow, but with a lower nutritional content.

Step 7: Clean (optional)

Place the fresh produce in a bowl of cold water and agitate gently, rinsing off any earth or debris if needed. Greens stay fresher if dried fully wrapped in a dry paper towel, then placed in an airtight container and refrigerated.

NOTES

- Consume greens as soon as possible after harvest, as compounds degrade through oxidization.

- Airflow is crucial for the health of the plants, and in reducing risk of mold and fruit fly issues. If there are no natural currents, fans serve well.

- Greens grow best in nutrient rich mediums with a moderate pH balance. It is wise to feed the soil or medium with nutritional powerhouses such as worm castings, rich compost, compost tea, or liquid kelp. After all, the nutrients will eventually build up in your own body.

- Growing mediums can be reused if kept clean and free of mucilaginous seeds like flax and chia. Mats can be boiled to clean and sterilize.

- If using topsoil, it would be of great benefit to start a vermicomposting set up to ensure proper cycling of organic matter.

MEDIUM OPTIONS

TOPSOIL

The most natural and basic Earth-centered material. Growing in topsoil allows the loving energy from our Mother Earth to manifest in the greens. Compositions vary dramatically between sources, consisting of components that retain water, provide drainage, and deliver nutrients. Topsoil can be messy and may create challenges with fungal and bacterial contamination. Choose a nutrient-rich soil with a high organic content (dark brown or black) and elements to reduce compaction such as peat, coir, vermiculite, or perlite.

VERMICULITE

Vermiculite is made from heat-expanded mica (a mined mineral) and is a common addition to potting soil. It is able to hold water and nutrients very well, and is best used for bigger seeds like grains, pea and sunflowers. It also boasts anti-fungal properties and delivers trace minerals, but is low in other nutrients such as nitrogen, phosphorus, and potassium. For this reason, it is advised to fertilize with a liquid-kelp product mixed into the irrigation water.

WORM CASTINGS

Organic matter digested by red wrigglers, worm castings are very high in nitrogen and is pathogen free; the magic of the worms transforms their food into highly valuable excrement. Exceptionally rich in humic acid, enzymes, and other beneficial life forms, worm castings are used as a nutritional additive (25% of the mixture) to soils or mediums that can feed leafy crops like sunflower. Helps with leaf development, flavor, and nutrition.

BABY BLANKET

This "blanket" is a felted plant-fiber mat made from jute or coconut, has decent moisture retention, and is especially well suited for clean cultivation of small seeds like brassicas. Void of nutrients, it is often supplemented with liquid kelp fertilizer. It can be sterilized and reused numerous times.

SURE-TO-GROW (STG)

Made from eucalyptus trees, STGs are used the same way as baby blankets.

COCONUT COIR (COY-ER)

Made from the outer husk of coconuts, this sustainable medium offers great moisture retention and brings an airy quality when used alone or as a mix. Offers slow mineral release and is often mixed with worm castings for added nutrition.

SPROUTING IN TRAYS

SMALL-SEEDED MICROGREENS

Any of the seeds that can be sprouted in jars or bags can also be planted in trays. For this method, the idea is to maintain moisture in the medium. As with a larger-scale environment, diversity is important and supports even, healthy growth. Mix seeds that have similar growth times and that balance each other out flavor-wise (for instance, blend sharp radish or broccoli with mild clover). It is best to soak and pre-sprout most seeds for 2 days or so to ensure more even and rapid growth with the exception of mucilaginous seeds such as cress, flax, and chia. Just be sure not to over soak brassicas as they can drown. For a standard 10 in x 20 in / 15 cm x 30 cm tray, plant about 4 tablespoons or ¼ C / 60 ml of seeds (dry volume).

ARUGULA (5 TO 14 DAYS)

Arugula is popular in salad mixes, and is just as flavorful and edgy as a micro green. Since the seeds are mucilaginous, plant them directly and do not soak.

BROCCOLI (5 TO 14 DAYS)

Broccoli has received considerable attention these days due to its high concentration of the antioxidant sulforaphane. These healing sprouts are full of bold, piquant flavor. Sprout before planting.

CABBAGE (5 TO 14 DAYS)

The deeply attractive purple cabbage sprouts are not only pretty, but also offer more concentrated nutrition than the mature plant. The downside is that sprouts are not so good for sauerkraut. Sprout before planting.

CHIA (5 TO 14 DAYS)

Not many people thought to eat their *Chia Pets*, but it's a great idea. Chia is gaining in popularity, and is high in omega-3 content. Plant directly and do not soak, as the seeds are mucilaginous.

LARGE-SEEDED MICROGREENS

These crops are on their way to becoming more like a garden crop, as they are more robust and larger in stature than small-seeded microgreens (except the ever-tender buckwheat). Soaked 8 to 15 hours and sprouted until the tails emerge (1 to 2 days), these larger seeds are easier to work with than smaller seeds: they are more forgiving, easier to plant, and less delicate to harvest. Sprouting before planting ensures consistent germination. Planting rates are 1½ C to 2 C / 350 ml to 500 ml dry volume (or 16 oz to 18 oz per standard 10-in x 20-in / 15-cm x 30-cm tray). Harvest before the second set of true leaves emerges.

BUCKWHEAT LETTUCE (7 TO 12 DAYS)

This microgreen has fragile and juicy stalks, as well as small, broad, and tender green leaves that unfold from triangular hulls. High in chlorophyll, vitamins A and C, calcium, lecithin, and rutin—a bioflavenoid that helps to eliminate excess cholesterol, increase blood circulation, and lower blood pressure. (Caution: Consume in moderation due to the presence of fagopyrin, a toxin that makes skin hypersensitive to light and creates uncomfortable tingling in the body—this condition is called fagopyrism. Note that buckwheat sprouts that have not reached the lettuce phase do not contain fagopyrin.)

SUNFLOWER GREENS (7 TO 12 DAYS)

These are scrumptious baby sunflowers with a crisp and nutty crunch. The smaller black oil seed (think birdseed) is better than the common larger type (used for eating whole as hulled seeds). The two thin, delicate leaves unfold when the shell is dropped, creating essential salad potential. High in chlorophyll, calcium, iron, phosphorous, lecithin, and vitamins B, D, and E.

POPCORN (8 TO 12 DAYS)

Wonderfully sweet sprouts can be grown from most popcorn seeds. By depriving the young shoots of light (blanching), the most tender and sweetest shoots are produced.

PEA SHOOTS (7 TO 12 DAYS)

Several different varieties of peas can grow young shoots that embody a mild green pea flavor with a perky stalk and subtle green leaves. Most commonly used is field pea or speckled pea. Very sweet and high in chlorophyll and vitamins A and C.

RECIPES

*Eat 'em on their own, eat 'em as a salad, eat 'em in smoothies, eat 'em
with soup, eat 'em in sandwiches, or eat 'em with entrees.
We can all use a little more green in our lives! And microgreens are a
superb addition to the diet. The possibilities are only limited by your
imagination, I'll offer a few suggestions here.*

GREEN SMOOTHIE

*This is an infinitely unique and delicious option. Whatever sprouts or
microgreens you have can combine well with numerous fruits, juices, and
seeds. Here is a guideline to get you started. Play around, have fun, and
enjoy the healthful creative process!*

INGREDIENTS

- 1 to 2 large handfuls microgreens

- 1 small handful sprouted seeds or nuts

- Juice, water, rejuvelac, or other liquid

PROCESS

Blend and ingest.

BASIC DRESSING

*This is an outline. From here, do whatever tickles your fancy. Fresh
ingredients are best minced finely, shredded, or blended with dressing.
Dress it up or down depending on your mood and what it's being paired
with. Try keeping it simple for sharp sprouts such as broccoli or fenugreek,
or use them to jazz up a softer flavor like pea shoots. If I like where the
dressing is headed, I'll make a bunch and keep it for later. Shake dressing
before serving since fat will separate (unless an emulsifier is added such as
mustard, flax, agar agar, or guar gum).*

INGREDIENTS

- 6 to 8 parts creamy (oil, nut butter in water, or thick mylk)

- 2 to 4 parts sour (lemon juice, apple cider vinegar, or balsamic vinegar)

- 1 to 2 parts sweet (honey, maple syrup, molasses, or agave syrup)

- Something savory (basil, rosemary, or cilantro)

- Something sharp (minced garlic, pepper, onion, or ginger)

- Something salty (tamari, salt, kelp, or miso)

PROCESS

Mix it up.

GREEN KALE SALAD

Pure, fresh, and simple. This salad is quick, easy, satisfying, and deeply nourishing.

INGREDIENTS

- ½ bunch kale
- 1 avocado
- 1 lemon, juiced
- Salt to taste

PROCESS

Take kale leaves in one hand and run the index finger and thumb of your other hand up each stem to separate the leaf from the stem. Tear the leaf into bite-size pieces. Massage kale to soften, and mix with microgreens. Dice avocado and dress with lemon juice.

SIMPLE SPINACH 'N SPROUTS

INGREDIENTS

- 2 large handfuls pea shoots
- 1 handful spinach
- ½ C / 125 ml lentil or pea sprouts
- 1 medium zucchini
- 2 Tbsp / 30 ml olive oil
- 2 Tbsp / 30 ml nutritional yeast
- 1 Tbsp / 15 ml apple cider vinegar
- 1 tsp / 5 ml tamari, shoyu, or Braggs liquid aminos
- A pinch of black pepper

PROCESS

Prepare zucchini in quartered coins, matchstick, or julienned (whatever your preference is). Tear spinach into bite-sized pieces, if needed, and add to sprouts and microgreens. Mix remaining ingredients in a cup, and then dress and enjoy.

ROOTS, SHOOTS, AND LEAVES

INGREDIENTS

- 3 to 4 carrots
- 1 large handful pea shoot and/or sunflower greens
- 1 handful greens (kale, arugula, or mesclun mix)
- ½ C / 125 ml lentil, mung, or pea sprouts
- ¼ C / 60 ml tahini or almond butter
- ¼ C / 60 ml water
- 3 Tbsp / 45 ml nutritional yeast
- 2 Tbsp / 30 ml apple cider vinegar
- 1 Tbsp / 15 ml honey, agave, or maple syrup
- 1 Tbsp / 15 ml miso
- 1 Tbsp / 15 ml ginger, shredded
- 1 clove of garlic, finely diced

PROCESS

Salad

If you have a mandolin, use it to julienne the carrots. Otherwise, cut carrots into matchstick shapes, or shred them. Roughly chop greens into bite-sized pieces, mix with sprouts, and set aside.

Sauce

Combine remaining ingredients together, and blend or shake vigorously. If shaking, start by mixing tahini and miso into a little water with a spoon. Once dissolved, mix in the rest and shake, shake, shake. Voila!

GROWING GRASS

It's quite alarming to think that we have forgotten the art of culturing our grains. The mechanized food system doesn't allow for germination to occur in the fields as it used to. The harvested sheaths being exposed to the elements were allowed to begin germinating, breaking down complex carbohydrates and activating vitamin and enzyme activity. Combine harvesters changed all that. Our systems have become too large to allow such rampant life force to run amok. Instead we control, sterilize, and strip the grains of their life force. But we are slowly remembering our roots through the local culturing of bread as sourdough gains popularity.

As a culture, we do not eat living grain. Instead, we ingest grain that is void of most life, sprayed with biocide poison, and possibly even irradiated. These processes are meant to protect us from spoiled or contaminated feed. After all, wheat in its whole, fresh, ground state can only last two weeks without refrigeration, as the oil in the germ goes rancid.

Grains have the advantage of naturally storing massive amounts of calories and nutrients in uniform units that can keep for years in the proper conditions. This also means this nutrition must be reawakened from its slumber in order to be of use to us. Not only are dry grains in a dormant state, but they also contain anti-nutrients like phytic acid, which are removed through sprouting and/or fermenting (see Neutralizing the Anti-Nutrients, page 26).

Many people all over the world know this, and it is reflected in their grain preparation. For example, take the common Middle Eastern dish bulgur—it's base is made of germinated, cracked, and dried wheat. Or take the Native American tradition of boiling corn with limestone (nixtamalization) to unlock nutrients, render corn much more digestible, and increase protein content. As agricultural societies evolved with grains, they learned the ways to make the best use of them.

Eating sprouted grains is a great way to get nutrition packed with fiber, enzymes (especially if left uncooked), trace elements, and vitamins (especially vitamin E). Sprouted grains can be added to cereals, tossed into soups (raw or cooked), made into breads and crackers (raw or cooked), and used as a base for beer malt or sweet syrups. Heartier grains, such as rye, kamut, spelt, barley, and wheat, can be steamed or cooked in a little water if a hot cereal is desired.

Think not what your grains can do for you, but what you can do for your grains.

CEREALS

WHEAT

Sweet and chewy, wheat is high in B vitamins, vitamin E, and a range of minerals. Gluten (a protein in wheat) is transformed through sprouting, and tends not to be an issue for many who are gluten sensitive (however, it is still an issue for celiacs). Make loaves by blending wheat in a food processor, shaping it, and then drying it in the sun or baking it. Make cream of wheat by adding water and blending. Try genetically diverse wheat varieties such as red fife or emmer.

BUCKWHEAT

This Central Asian pseudograin (containing two cotyledons) is soft, mild, and slightly nutty. Buckwheat is unrelated to wheat, making it 100% gluten free. The seeds, or groats, are very easily digested and contain a complete protein profile, high amounts of vitamins A and C, calcium, and rutin. Make sure not to oversoak and to rinse well as seeds create mucilage (viscous, pinkish liquid) when soaked. Sprouted buckwheat can be dehydrated in a dehydrator, or an oven set at the lowest temp for 12 to 24 hours (until crispy).

OATS

The best oats to sprout are hulless oats, as opposed to the common variety that requires dehulling. Oats are high in soluble fiber, protein, and fat (and are one the of highest sources of these among grains). Whole groats can be soaked (12 to 48 hours to soften and deactivate enzyme inhibitors called phytates) and eaten raw, allowed to ferment, and/or cooked. Rolled oats soften very quickly and create delightful creaminess when soaked in just water.

I have chosen not to include recipes using sprouted flour—a shelf-stable product produced by Essential Eating Sprouted Food (see Resources, page 124)—because I want to focus on what the average home sprouter can do with his/her sprouted seeds. For the record, I do support the use of such products.

SPROUTING GRAINS

The young stages of cereal grass development provide some of the most nutrient dense juice on the planet. They are host to an incredible array of minerals, a complete range of essential amino acids, and chlorophyll. Along with spirulina (blue-green algae, or cyanobacteria) and chlorella (green algae), these grasses are also among a select few foods that contain the nucleic acids RNA and DNA, which can defend the body against radiation.

By absorbing and synthesizing nutrients from the soil and sun, and storing them in the young grass blades, these grasses offer readily available nutrients when consumed. Chewing or juicing grasses is required for us to reap the nutritional benefits from them, unlike ruminants (such as cows) that can digest the rough cellulosic fiber.

Consuming grass juice is an excellent way to alkalize the body, balance blood-sugar levels, reduce inflammation, cleanse the blood, improve digestion, lower blood pressure, and deodorize the body. These benefits are derived from the abundance of enzymes, chlorophyll, vitamins, and minerals naturally present in young grass. The high oxygen content of the juice has a beneficial effect on overall rejuvenation and promotes youthfulness.

Grasses are planted in the same manner as microgreens—sprout before planting, and then plant densely at 2 C to 4 C / 500 ml to 1000 ml of seed per standard 10-in x 20-in / 15-cm x 30-cm tray.

WHEATGRASS (7 TO 10 DAYS)

By far, wheatgrass is the most popular of the cereal grasses to grow. The juice is distinctly deep green and sweet in a complex way. One ounce provides a wealth of amino acids, enzymes, 92 of the 102 essential minerals (mainly calcium, phosphorus, iron, magnesium, and potassium), and vitamins A, B, C, E, and K. Hard wheat is used.

SPELT AND KAMUT GRASSES (7 TO 10 DAYS)

These are ideal ancient alternatives to wheat due to their lack of hybridization. They are very similar to wheat in sweetness with a slightly bitter twang. Viable seeds may be harder to come by.

BARLEY GRASS (7 TO 10 DAYS)

Slightly more bitter than wheat, owing to a more diverse mineral portfolio. Be sure to obtain whole "sprouting barley," as many barley products won't sprout.

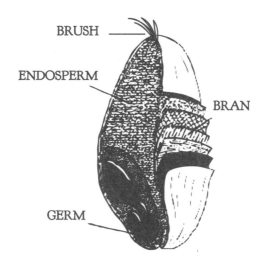

BRUSH

ENDOSPERM

BRAN

GERM

RECIPES

APPLE CINNAMON BREAKFAST BOWL

This dish can be prepared ahead of time for a quick and easy breakfast for two. This meal is thoroughly delicious, full of antioxidants and omega-3s, and is satisfying without being too heavy.

INGREDIENTS

- ½ C / 125 ml sprouted buckwheat
- ½ C / 125 ml sprouted quinoa
- ¼ C / 60 ml sunflower seeds or almonds, soaked
- 2 Tbsp / 60 ml ground flax
- 1 apple, finely diced
- 2 tsp / 10 ml cinnamon
- 1 tsp / 5 ml cardamom
- 1 Tbsp / 15 ml maple syrup or honey (optional)
- 1 ½ C / 375 ml mylk of choice (hemp is my favorite)

PREPARATION:

Simply mix all ingredients together.

SIMPLE MUESLI

A European breakfast staple. This simple dish is eaten cold and is a delightful summer breakfast. Soaking reduces phytic acid in the grains.

INGREDIENTS

- ½ C / 125 ml rolled oats or other grain
- ¼ C / 60 ml pumpkin and/or sunflower seed
- ¼ C / 60 ml raisins or other dried fruit
- Mylk or yogurt to cover (optional)

PROCESS

Combine rolled oats, fruit, and water in a bowl with enough water to cover overnight. Soak seeds in separate container. Drain and rinse seeds in the morning, and then mix all together.

BASIC GRAWNOLA

*This base recipe is a satisfying raw version of a common cereal snack.
Grawnola can be dressed up however you like by tossing in fruits and
varying the spices, and can be served with different mylks or smoothies.*

INGREDIENTS

- 2 C / 500 ml sprouted (12 to 36 hours) buckwheat
- 1 ½ C / 375 ml combo of soaked seeds/nuts
- ¼ C / 60 ml ground flax seed
- 1/2 C / 120 ml honey, maple syrup, or agave
- 2 Tbsp / 60 ml coconut or olive oil
- 1 Tbsp / 15 ml vanilla extract, or 1 vanilla bean
- 1 Tbsp / 15 ml cinnamon
- 1 tsp / 5 ml nutmeg
- ¼ tsp / 1.25 ml sea salt

PROCESS

You can choose to eat it fresh, but crunchy is really where it's at. If drying
it, be sure the sprouts are well drained. Mix moist ingredients together
well before adding them to sprouts, and then mix by hand. Spread evenly
on dehydrator sheets and dry at 100°F / 37°C for 12 to 24 hours. If not
available, use baking pans and put in oven with the light on. Or heat using
the lowest setting, or by placing mixture in the warming tray until crispy.

VARIATIONS

By using the above recipe as a guideline, the options are unlimited. Be
inspired! It's important to flow with your preferences, and with what
you have on hand. The nuts/seeds listed in the recipes can be used
interchangeably.

APPLE WALNUT

- 2 medium apples
- 1 C / 250 ml soaked sunflower seeds
- ½ C / 125 ml soaked walnut
- 3 tsp / 15 ml fresh ginger, shredded (or 2 tsp / 10 ml powdered)

BLUEBERRY BLISS

- 1 C / 250 ml fresh blueberries
- 1 C / 250 ml coconut, shredded or flaked

CHOCO CRUNCH

- 1 C / 250 ml soaked and rough cut cashews
- ½ C / 125 ml soaked almonds
- ½ C / 125 ml raw cacao nibs
- ¼ C / 60 ml raw cacao powder

ALMOND 'N' APRICOT

- 1 C / 250 ml almonds
- ½ C / 125 ml pumpkin seeds
- 1 C / 125 ml unsulphured apricots, diced
- 1 tsp / 5 ml almond extract

ESSENE BREAD (A.K.A. MANA BREAD)

Some recipe instructions are provided in an excerpt from The Essene
Gospel of Peace. *This work was translated from the* Dead Sea Scrolls
*and offer guidance for making bread. The Essences were an ancient Jewish
mystical sect, of which Jesus was a part for a time, that were focused on
living healthy, selfless, and pure lives.*

*"Let the angels of God prepare your bread. Moisten your wheat, that the
angel of water may enter it. Then set it in the air, that the angel of air
also may embrace it. And leave it from morning to evening beneath the
sun, that the angel of sunshine may descend upon it. And the blessing of
the three angels will soon make the germ of life to sprout in your wheat.
Then crush your grain and make thin wafers, as did your forefathers when
they departed out of Egypt, the house of bondage. Put them back again
beneath the sun from its appearing and when it is risen to its highest in the
heavens, turn them over on the other side that they be embraced there also
by the angel of sunshine and leave them there until the sun be set..."*
Makes 2 medium loaves.

INGREDIENTS

- 2 C / 500 ml dry kamut, spelt, wheat, or rye

- ½ tsp / 2.5 ml salt

- 1 C / 250 ml raisins (soaked 30 mins)

- 2 medium carrots

- 2 Tbsp / 30m ml coconut or olive oil (maintain pliability)

- 2 Tbsp / 30 ml pure water (as little water as possible, start with less and add
more if needed to form loaves)

PROCESS

Step 1: Sprout

Soak, drain, and sprout the grain for 2 days, until the tail is as long as the seed.

Step 2: Grind

Grind the grain in a hand mill, high-powered blender, or food processor in successive batches.

Step 3: Mix

Mix other ingredients together with dough. Add additional ingredients little by little.

Step 4: Shape

Shape with wet hands (prevents sticking) into desired shape, making sure it's of consistent thickness to ensure consistent drying.

Step 5: Dry

Dry under the sun or in a dehydrator, or bake in the oven. If using the sun, pray for a sunny day and place outside on a rock or screen, following the instructions from *The Essene Gospel of Peace*. If using a dehydrator, place bread on a nonstick sheet for 4 hours, before removing sheet and flipping. Continue drying for about 24 hours until desired texture is reached. If using the oven, bake at 160°F to 250°F/ 70°C to 120°C until bread has reached desired texture. Bake time depends on temperature and thickness. You can heat it in the oven for 1 to 2 hours, turn off the oven, and then leave the bread to bake in the residual heat.

NOTE

Fruit and vegetables aren't needed, but can add a nice touch of sweetness and texture. Add apple, date, beet, onion, or whatever tickles your fancy.

RYE-VITAL CRACKERS

Play around with this recipe: substitute in other grains and seeds, and toss in different herbs or seasonal greens like dandelion or nettles. The combinations are unlimited.

INGREDIENTS

- 2 C / 500 ml rye grain
- 1 ½ C / 375 ml pure water
- 2 cloves of raw garlic
- 1 Tbsp / 15 ml caraway or cumin seeds
- 1 tsp / 5 ml high-quality salt
- ½ tsp / 2.5 ml black pepper, freshly ground

PREPARATION

Step 1: Sprout

Sprout rye until tails are as long as the seed (2 days or so).

Step 2: Grind

Grind sprouts in a hand mill, high-powered blender, or food processor in successive batches. Add other ingredients in proportion to the sprouts.

Step 3: Spread

Spread thinly and evenly on nonstick sheets or parchment paper. Mixture should be about ¼ in / 0.6 cm thick.

Step 4: Dry

Dry in dehydrator for 4 hours, remove sheet, and flip. Dry another 4 hours or until crispy. If using the oven, place on cookie sheets or baking pans, and use oven light or lowest heat setting to dry, which preserves enzymes. Dry until crispy.

REJUVELAC

This is a refreshing enzyme rich beverage popularized by Dr. Ann Wigmore,
who was famous for her work with healing serious and chronic illnesses
with living foods. Rejuvelac helps balance the body's pH while providing
hydration and essential nutrients. It is a slightly fermented beverage that
contains all the nutrients of the grain from which it was cultured (complex
B vitamins, as well as C and E). Available probiotic bacteria help promote
healthy flora in the GI tract and aids in the elimination of toxins in the
colon. It can be made with wheat, rye, millet, quinoa, or any other grain
or pseudo-grain (each with their own character and profile). My personal
favorite is quinoa. A great way to begin the day is with a lukewarm glass
of rejuvelac to awaken the system and prepare the stomach for digestion.
Adapted from Sally Fallon's Nourishing Traditions.

MATERIALS

- Raw, organic, sproutable grain

- Filtered or purified water

- Large (1 Quart / 1 Liter) glass jar

- Screen (or sprouting lid)

PROCESS
Step 1: Soak

Place ½ C grains in 1-Q / 1-L jar and rinse grain before covering with three
times as much water to soak. Secure the lid or sprouting screen and soak
for 8 to 15 hours.

Step 2: Drain

Pour off water, but do not rinse (normally done when sprouting). Leave sprouts without rinsing for 2 days until small tails appear as long as the grain.

Step 3: Ferment

Fill the jar with water and let ferment 24 to 72 hours at room temperature.

Step 4: Strain

Strain off grain and pour Rejuvelac into a separate jar, and then store in a sealed container in the fridge. It will keep for several days. The leftover grain can be used to ferment another batch of Rejuvelac up to three times.

NOTE

The longer it is left to ferment, the stronger the Rejuvelac will taste. It should be slightly tart (similar to citrus), cloudy, and have a slighty yellow tint. Tiny bubbles will occur (natural carbonation) due to fermentation, and a thin layer of foam may develop. The smell is strange, even offensive at first, but the taste is much more agreeable and mild. Quinoa seems to make the best Rejuvelac in my opinion. It will keep in the fridge for about a week. Leftover grain can be eaten raw, cooked as usual, made into bread or crackers, or fed to pets.

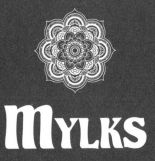

Mylks

Non-dairy mylks can be made from fatty seeds, nuts, and oats. These mylks take the strain off cows, the environment, and our bodies (by avoiding difficult to digest lactose, growth hormones, and antibiotics). While there are commercially available alternatives to milk (soy, almond, and rice milks), these options are all pasteurized (heated to high temperatures), which destroys enzymes. These products cost more to make, and are also energy intensive to produce, package, store, and transport.

By making your own mylk at home, you can be sure that you have a vibrantly alive, cost-effective, and environmentally friendly product. And homemade mylks can be used in the same ways as commercial varieties!

HEMP

Scrumptiously nutty and creamy, hemp is the most sustainable of the seeds due to its independence from fertilizers, herbicides, or pesticides. The hulled seeds, or hemp hearts, boast a full range of essential fatty acids in balanced proportions (omega-3, 6, and 9), and is a rich source of calcium, iron, magnesium, and potassium. Since hemp contains all of the essential amino acids, it's considered to be a complete protein. It also contains a plant protein (edestin) that is as easily digestible as proteins found in mother's milk.

Note: Most hemp is sold as "hearts" with shells removed. These are not to be drained if soaked. Whole hemp seeds can be sprouted and made into mylk, but must be strained (the result has a short shelf life).

SUNFLOWER

Raw, hulled sunflower seeds are the most economical of the seeds. Native to North America, sunflowers have been grown, and their seeds eaten, by North Americans for centuries. Hulled seeds are widely available, and are high in protein, thiamin, vitamin B6, magnesium, manganese, selenium, and vitamin E. These seeds are mild and adaptable, and are the quickest of all the mylk-making seeds to ferment once blended. Like the flesh of apples, sunflower seed go brown when exposed to air (oxidization).

ALMOND

A tree crop native to the Middle East and South Asia, almonds are related to plums, apricots, and cherries. Almonds are traditionally eaten as a snack out of hand, and also serve as a base for curries and sweets. They are a great source of protein, B vitamins, fiber, magnesium, copper, manganese, potassium, and calcium. Almond skins can irritate the GI tract, so remove them if you so desire—pinching or squeezing them between fingers will make them slide off easily after soaking. As of 2007, forced pasteurization of almonds from California has brought into question the "raw" state of U.S. almonds.

RECIPES

BASIC MYLK

MATERIALS

- Raw, organic seeds (sunflower, pumpkin, sesame, etc.) or nuts (almond, cashew, etc.)

- Blender, food processor, or pestle and mortar

- Nut-mylk or sprout bag*, cheesecloth, or metal strainer (optional)

  *Tightly woven, food-grade nylon sacks are sold for this purpose.

INGREDIENTS

- ½ C / 125 ml seeds or nuts

- 1 ½ C to 2 C / 375 ml to 500 ml water

- A pinch of sea salt (optional)

- Sweetener: honey, maple syrup, fruit, or stevia (optional)

- Spices or other flavorings such as vanilla, cinnamon, or turmeric (optional)

PROCESS

Step 1: Soak

Soak seeds or nuts for their respective times (overnight is adequate).

Step 2: Rinse

Pour off water, and rinse well with clean water to wash away anti-nutrients.

Step 3: Blend

Add ½ C / 125 ml fresh water along with seeds or nuts in a blending device, and blend at high speed until creamy. It should be thick (consistency allows for more thorough blending). If using mortar or grinder, don't add water.

Step 4: Dilute

Add remainder of water until desired consistency is reached, which depends on your preference and intended use.

Step 5: Strain (optional)

Pour contents into bag, cheesecloth, or metal strainer. Squeeze as much of the liquid out as possible. The pulp can be used for cookies, crackers, or breads.

Step 6: Season

Blend in optional ingredients

NOTES

- Mylks keep in fridge for several days (up to a week). Left out, they will ferment, which you may like.

- Unless you're adding an emulsifier like flax or guar gum, solids and liquid will separate naturally. Just stir mylk before serving.

- Mylks can also be made from oats and pseudo-grains, such as quinoa and buckwheat, using a water ratio of 2:1.

GOLDEN MYLK

A variation on an Indian classic. This drink is warming, grounding, and helps reduce inflammation, thanks to the turmeric.

INGREDIENTS

- 2 C to 3 C / 500 ml to 750 ml water

- ½ C sesame, sunflower, or pumpkin seeds

- 1 tsp / 5 ml turmeric powder

- ½ tsp / 2.5 ml cinnamon or nutmeg

- ¼ tsp / 1.25 ml black pepper, ground

- Sweetener of choice, if desired

PROCESS

Step 1: Soak

Soak seeds according to chart.

Step 2: Drain

Thoroughly wash soaked seeds.

Step 3: Blend, Dilute and Strain

Follow the instructions for basic Mylk, steps 3 through 5 on page 94.

Step 5: Heat and Season

Pour mylk into pot and heat slowly while stirring in the seasonings. Heat until warm (but not boiling) and drink.

HORCHATA

*A refreshing beverage from Mexico that's traditionally made with tiger nuts
and honey, but that's popularly made with cow's milk, white sugar, and
white rice seasoned with cinnamon and vanilla. Served cold and garnished
with cinnamon, horchata is light and satisfying.*

INGREDIENTS

- 4 C / 1 L water
- ½ C / 125 ml raw almonds
- 2 Tbsp to 4 Tbsp / 30 ml to 60 ml honey, agave, or maple syrup (to taste)
- 1 tsp / 5 ml vanilla extract, or ½ vanilla bean (use insides only)
- ½ tsp / 2.5 ml true cinnamon powder (a.k.a. Saigon cinnamon)

PROCESS

Step 1: Soak

Soak almonds 8 to 12 hours.

Step 2: Drain

Thoroughly wash soaked almonds. Remove skins, if desired.

Step 3: Blend

Add almonds and ½ C / 125 ml water and blend, slowly adding water.

Step 4: Strain

Place in bag or cheesecloth and squeeze as much of the liquid out as possible.
Use pulp for cookies, crackers, or breads.

Step 5: Season

Add remaining ingredients and sweeten to taste. Serve chilled with a
sprinkling of cinnamon to garnish.

XOCOLATL

Originally, chocolate was consumed as a drink by members of the royalty in Mesoamerica. Xocolatl (the word for chocolate in the indigenous language of Náhuatl) translates as "bitter water," and started out as a bitter medicinal drink, not a sweet candy. The beverage has a base of ground corn and cacao, inviting additions of vanilla, cinnamon, chilies, bee pollen, and honey. Here's a new spin on an ancient beverage.

INGREDIENTS

- 2 C / 500 ml mylk
- ¼ C / 60 ml carob or cacao powder (the purest raw form of cocoa)
- 2 Tbsp to 4 Tbsp / 30 ml to 60 ml honey, agave, or maple syrup
- 2 Tbsp / 60 ml coconut oil or cocoa butter
- ½ tsp / 2.5 ml vanilla extract, or ¼ vanilla bean
- ⅛ tsp to ¼ tsp / 0.5 ml to 1 ml chipotle or other chilies, to taste
- A pinch of salt

PROCESS

Mix and drink.

DOSHA BALANCING DRINK

The ancient system of Ayurveda seeks to balance an individual's constitution, or dosha. This drink combination is said to balance all three doshas. A warming base of nourishing sesame and pungent spices help to balance the cooling sweet fruit. The spices have a soothing effect on the nerves and digestion as well.

INGREDIENTS

- 2 C / 500 ml sesame milk
- 1 banana
- 1 Tbsp to 2 Tbsp / 30 ml to 60 ml honey or maple syrup, or 5 juicy dates
- ½ tsp / 2.5 ml cardamom
- ½ tsp / 2.5 ml cinnamon
- ¼ tsp / 1.25 ml turmeric
- A pinch of salt

PROCESS

Mix and drink.

CREAMY CIDER

- 2 C / 500 ml apple cider
- ¼ C hemp seeds or cashews
- 1 tsp / 5 ml ginger, freshly grated
- 1 tsp / 5 ml cinnamon
- ½ tsp / 2.5 ml cloves

PROCESS
Mix and drink.

BERRY BLAST MYLKSHAKE

- 2 C / 500 ml mylk
- ¾ C / 175 ml fresh or frozen berries
- ½ C / 125 ml raw spinach
- 1 Tbsp to 2 Tbsp / 15 ml to 30 ml honey or maple syrup (optional)

PROCESS
Mix and drink.

Non-Dairy Cultures

This section opens up a range of possibilities and flavors. Although scrumptious, these non-dairy cultures do not behave like their dairy counterparts. Comparatively, they will not keep for long periods of time like some dairy products, nor will they melt in the same manner. Nevertheless, these products are delicious, nutritious, versatile, and more economically sound in terms of production than many dairy products.

Cultured foods, such as "cheeses" or "yogurts," can be made by fermenting seeds or nuts that have first been blended and sprouted; this can be done with or without a starter culture. These cultures speed up the processing time and ensure more thorough and even fermentation, but are not necessary by nature. Nuts and seeds in this state are very easily digested, and the nutrients are quickly assimilated and offer probiotics, which are a result of lactic-acid- producing bacteria tbat act to balance pH and to kill invading microbes while restoring beneficial microbes in our bodies. Therefore, lactic acid and enzymes produced through fermentation greatly benefit metabolism, increase digestive health, and help boost immunity.

Variations on recipe bases can be created using fruits and vegetables to add texture, flavor, color, and nutrition. Yogurts can be made especially exquisite with blueberries or pears. Cheeses are enhanced by these complementary ingredients: garlic, onion, beets, nettles, and seaweeds such as kelp or dulse (soft and very rich in minerals).

Different seeds and nuts offer different options and results. For example, almonds and sunflower seeds make neutral yet delicious cultures, hemp and pumpkin seeds create a full-body, nutty experience, while cashews provide a decadently velvet-like smoothness. This realm is truly one of experimentation, so have fun and play around with variations as you see fit.

RECIPES

BASIC CHEESE

INGREDIENTS

- 2 C / 500 ml soaked nuts or seeds*

- ½ C to 1 C / 125 ml to 250 ml Rejuvelac**

OR

- ½ C to 1 C / 125 ml to 250 ml water + 2 tsp / 10 ml miso

- ¼ C / 60 ml nutritional yeast

- 2 Tbsp / 60 ml apple cider vinegar, or juice of half a lemon (optional, helps to prevent oxidative discoloration)

    *Any combination can be used.

    **Another option is kombucha. If nothing of the sort is available, water will work. However, it will take a little longer and may be less consistent as it is a fully wild ferment.

PROCESS
Step 1: Blend
Blend all ingredients together with just enough Rejuvelac or water until a smooth, thick paste is achieved. A few chunks are okay and may be desired for texture. Place contents in a glass jar. Any leftover liquid can be set aside for other usage.

Step 2: Ferment
Cover jar with a clean towel or cloth and leave at room temperature for 8 to 48 hours. Fermentation time depends on temperature, desired taste, and

consistency. The cheese will separate from the liquid once fermented and will smell slightly tangy.

Step 3: Strain and Age

Pour through cheesecloth, sprout bag, or strainer, wringing out as much liquid as possible—the drier, the better. Browning may occur (oxidization); this is normal.

Step 4: Store

You may choose to mold the cheese into appealing shapes before serving. By placing it in sealed jar, the cheese will keep in fridge for up to 5 days, although it rarely does because it's just so delicious.

NOTES

Cheeses do not need to drain and can be simply used as is. Straining does create a nice density and presentation. See directions in Spicy Seed Cheese Recipe on the next page. Another option for texture is to add agar agar (a seaweed) to the cheese to thicken and bind it, and to make it more suitable for cutting.

SPICY SEED CHEESE

Adapted from Almond Essence *by Janet L. Doane*

INGREDIENTS

- ½ C / 125 ml pumpkin seeds
- ½ C / 125 ml sunflower seeds
- ¼ C Rejuvelac or water
- ¼ C / 60 ml nutritional yeast
- 2 Tbsp / 60 ml lemon, lime, or apple cider vinegar
- 1 small clove of garlic, peeled, and minced
- 1 tsp / 5 ml cumin powder
- ½ tsp / 2.5 ml paprika
- ½ tsp / 2.5 ml sea salt
- ¼ tsp / 1.25 ml chipotle powder

PROCESS

Step 1: Sprout

Soak seeds 4 to 12 hours, and then rinse and drain as usual.

Step 2: Puree

Place all ingredients in a food processor or high-powered blender, and puree until smooth.

Step 3: Age

Place mixture in mylk bag, or cheesecloth, and form into a ball, compressing the side to expel liquid. Hang above a bowl to catch drips and allow maturation in a warm place for 3 days or more.

Step 4: Store

Once mature enough by taste, you can mold cheese and add a sprinkling of paprika if desired. Or simply store in airtight container in the fridge.

....

GOURMET MEDITERRANEAN CHEESE

INGREDIENTS

- 1 C / 250 ml raw cashews
- ¼ C / 60 ml nutritional yeast
- ¼ C / 60 ml kombucha tea or water with 1 tsp / 5 ml miso
- 1 Tbsp fresh lemon juice or apple cider vinegar
- 1 tsp / 5 ml salt
- 1 tsp / 5 ml black pepper
- 2 Tbsp / 30 ml fresh rosemary, chopped
- 2 Tbsp / 30 ml basil or thyme

PROCESS

Same as Spicy Seed Cheese, page 105.

YOGURT

INGREDIENTS

- 1 C / 250 ml seeds or nuts
- 2 ¼ C / 560 ml water
- Starter culture powder, ¼ C to ½ C / 60 ml to 125 ml commercial yogurt, or 1 probiotic tablet
- Thickening agent:

    ⸗Ground flax seed, chia, arrowroot powder, tapioca flour: Dissolve 3 Tbsp / 45 ml in a little water before mixing.

    ⸗Guar gum: Add 1 tsp to 2 tsp / 5 ml to 10 ml in a little water before mixing.

    ⸗Agar agar powder (a seaweed) or xantham gum: Add ½ tsp to 1 tsp

    ⸗Liquid Lecithin: Add ¼ tsp / 1.25 ml

- Flavorings and/or fruits (optional)

PROCESS

Step 1: Blend

Blend mylk as usual until smooth. Straining is a matter of texture preference.

Step 2: Thicken

This step can help create a fuller-bodied yogurt, but may not be desired if unstrained mylk is used. Thickening will also help emulsify, and stop liquids and solids from separating. Pick a thickener or combine those listed above.

Step 3: Culture

Some sources recommend bringing mylk to boil, but this is not necessary. The culture will not survive at boiling temperatures, so make sure the mylk is cool enough to keep your finger submerged, and comfortably hot to the touch, between 90°F and 115°F/32°C and 46°C. Pitch the starter and mix well into the mylk. Pour into jars warmed in hot water, and place in a closed oven with the light left on. Cover jars with a cloth or towel to maintain 110°F/43°C for 6 to 9 hours (the longer, the sourer).

NOTES

If the yogurt falls short on texture, do not worry; it will still be healthy. Pay closer attention to temperature and try another starter option. Err on the side of too little starter, as the resulting yogurt will taste too strong and may turn out soupy. If liquids and solids separate, just stir them together before eating.

Conclusion

The intention of this manual is to awaken an interest in sprouting, and to be a reminder of the beauty of natural processes and the resulting potential to thrive. An earnest effort and a subtle shift are all that is required to incorporate sprouting into your daily life, and to nourish your body with the life forces of seeds. Sprouting can be a lifelong passion, and serve to maintain and promote vitality and wellness through caring for self and seeds.

Sprouting was first introduced to me in 2006 in Nova Scotia on one of the many farms at which I spent time as a WWOOF (World Wide Opportunities on Organic Farms) intern. I picked up the book *Survival into the 21st Century: Planetary Healers* by Viktoras Kulvinskas and was enthralled by the idea that I could enhance my own food already in my pantry through sprouting and have a dramatically positive effect on my health in doing so. Since that time, I've been sprouting non-stop.

I've brought my EASY SPROUT™ with me on my travels around the world and am always sharing sprouts with the folks I meet. Most find it odd at first to see a little bin being taken from my backpack with sprouted lentils in it, but EASY SPROUT™ is a durable, food-grade HDPE plastic container that uses convection to aerate the growing sprouts. I recommend it as a tool in sprouting; it is very easy to use and carry, requires little water, and has served me personally on many voyages from trains to back country expeditions.

I've since eaten in dozens of kitchens in several countries and shared food over many languages. What has touched me the most is a common thread of unified humanity and the power that sprouted foods hold in enhancing holistic health worldwide. In sharing this approach to sprouted foods with those I meet, I am sharing a part of myself, just as I am learning about another culture's wisdom.

Sprouting has offered me so much more than good nutrition. It has become a gateway into nature's enigma, a peek into the miracle of life, and an invitation to dine with Mother Earth.

Once sprouting has become a part of your life, try saving your own seeds from your garden to complete the cycles of birth and rebirth. Brassicas produce copious seeds their second year of growth and can be easily harvested and stored for year-round sprouts. This offers a tangible element of a sustainable and resilient lifestyle. In an ever-changing world, having some degree of self-sufficiency is highly valauble. By learning how to sprout, you are taking more responsibility for your food and life source. Happy sprouting!

GLOSSARY

ANTI-CARCINOGEN: Used to describe a substance or compound that inhibits the growth of cancerous cells either by deactivating carcinogens, or by blocking their mechanisms of action.

ANTI-NUTRIENT: Any substance that inhibits or interferes with the nutrient absorption process. Present in plants to inhibit consumption or premature germination.

ANTIOXIDANT: A molecule that prevents oxidative damage to cells, and is also able to neutralize free radicals in order to protect the body.

ASAFOETIDA: *Ferula assa-foetida* is an herb in the Apiaceae family (celery, dill, etc.) that's used as an Indian seasoning to flavor and harmonize dishes. It also has the ability to increase the digestibility of legumes while reducing flatulence.

BIOAVAILABILITY: The capacity for life forms to utilize and access certain compounds.

BIOGENIC: Referring to foods that are living and are able to transmit the energy within themselves to consumers.

BRASSICA: Members of the Brassicaceae or Cruciferea family such as broccoli, kale, cabbage, cress, and mustard.

CANAVANINE: A toxin that is present in seeds to protect for herbivorous consumption, present in very low concentrations in alfalfa and other legumes.

CEREAL: A synonym for grains or monocot seeds.

CHELATE: Refers to mineral ions bound to proteins, a bioavailable form of minerals found in sprouts.

CHLOROPHYLL: Green pigment in leaves and algaes, attracting sunlight and thereby enabling photosynthesis. Especially important for human health due to its detoxifying, oxygenating and blood cleansing effects.

COTYLEDON: Also known as seed leaves, cotyledons are the first leaves to emerge from a seed and are used as a food supply for a germinating embryo.

DICOT: A flowering plant with two cotyledons, such as buckwheat and quinoa.

EDESTIN: Easily digestible plant protein found in hemp hearts that is similar to proteins found in mother's milk.

ENZYME: Molecules that act as catalysts for reactions in the body. Highly selective in their function, and part of the metabolic processes that serve to maintain life. The presence of enzymes is an important part of longevity and vitality.

ENZYME INHIBITOR: Anti-nutritive substances found in seeds designed to stop germination and to deter predators. Soaking and rinsing the seeds before consumption eliminates the potential for the negative effects they may impose on our bodies.

EPAZOTE: Native to Central and South America, *Dysphania ambrosioides* is a bitter plant belonging to the Amaranthaceae family. Epazote is popularly used to flavor bean dishes, due to its pungent flavor, and its ability to reduce flatulence and to make beans more digestible.

FREE RADICAL: Unstable molecule capable of damaging cellular DNA.

GERM: The reproductive part of a seed containing the embryo and chromosomes.

GERMINATION: The waking up and initial growth process of a seed; the first step in becoming a plant.

GROAT: A seed whose hull has been removed. Buckwheat and oats both are sold as groats. Buckwheat groats can be sprouted whereas oats cannot unless a variety of hulless oats is used.

HULL: The protective outer coating of a seed.

HULLED: Referring to seeds that have had their hulls removed mechanically.

ISOFLAVONES: A class of organic compounds found almost exclusively in plants in the Fabaceae family that have antioxidant activity, and that influence sex hormones, protein syntheses, and other biological activities.

LEGUME: A plant in the Fabaceae family, commonly known as the pea family. Classified by its ability to fix nitrogen in the soil utilizing nodes on its roots and symbiotic fungi. Well-known legumes include lentils, chickpeas, peas, alfalfa, and clover.

LIGNANS: A class of organic compounds known as phytoestrogens that are found in plants; they have both estrogenic and antioxidant activity.

METHYLATION: A process affecting gene expression involving the addition of a methyl group (CH_3) to a DNA base. It is responsible for most vital aspects of body chemistry, and allows us to be healthy and vital.

MICROGREENS: Seeds grown with a medium.

MONOCOT: A flowering plant with one cotyledon. True cereals, such as wheat and rice, are monocots.

MUCILAGE: A thick, glue-like substance produced by plants. Used to trap and conserve moisture during germination. Once moistened, seeds such as flax, chia, cress, and (to a lesser extent) buckwheat become mucilaginous.

PATHOGEN: Anything that can cause disease or infection such as salmonella or *E.coli*.

PHASEOLUS GENUS: A category of beans in the Fabaceae family, all of which are native to North America

PHOTOSYNTHESIS: The conversion of sunlight into energy in the form of sugars by plants, algae, and cyanobacteria.

PHYTIC ACID: An anti-nutrient found in grains, nuts, and seeds. Responsible for decreasing digestibility, lowering bioavailability, increasing risk of cavities, and imposing other detrimental effects on the body. It is removed by soaking, sprouting, and/or fermenting foods.

PHYTOCHEMICAL: Chemicals produced by plants as a defense or protection mechanism. Phytonutrients are included in this group.

PHYTONUTRIENT: A chemical compound produced in plants that are of nutritional and medicinal value to humans.

PLUMULE: The underdeveloped primary shoot within a seed.

POLYPHENOLS: A class of chemicals occurring in plants, often with protective properties for the plants as well as our bodies. There are various names for the different polyphenols as well as distinct actions when eaten.

PSEUDOGRAIN: A seed that may resemble or share uses with cereal grains (see Monocot), but belonging to another group of plants (see Dicot) such as quinoa and buckwheat. These seeds are all gluten free.

RADICLE: Young root emerging from a germinating seed. Also referred to in this book as "tails."

SHOOT: Another name for microgreens grown from peas and sunflowers.

VERMICOMPOST: A nutrient-cycling system most often using red wrigglers as the convertors of food scraps into worm castings.

WORM CASTINGS: A very useful soil amendment with high nutrient content and beneficial chemicals such as humic and fulvic acid.

SPROUTING
CHART

ADZUKI	*8 HRS SOAKING*	*3 TO 5 DAYS SPROUTING*	
ALFALFA	*8 HRS SOAKING*	*2 TO 5 DAYS SPROUTING*	
ALMOND	*8 TO 12 HRS SOAKING*	*½ TO 3 DAYS SPROUTING*	
BARLEY	*6 TO 12 HRS SOAKING*	*2 TO 3 DAYS SPROUTING*	
BRAZILNUT	*DOES NOT SOAK*	*DOES NOT SPROUT*	
BUCKWHEAT	*15 MIN SOAKING*	*6 HRS SPROUTING*	
CASHEW	*2 TO 2½ HRS SOAKING*	*DOES NOT SPROUT*	
CHICKPEA	*12 HRS SOAKING*	*2 TO 3 DAYS SPROUTING*	
CORN	*12 HRS SOAKING*	*2 TO 3 DAYS SPROUTING*	
FENUGREEK	*8 HRS SOAKING*	*3 TO 5 DAYS SPROUTING*	
FLAX	*8 HRS SOAKING*	*DOES NOT SPROUT*	
HEMP	*DOES NOT SOAK*	*DOES NOT SPROUT*	
KAMUT	*7 HRS SOAKING*	*2 TO 3 DAYS SPROUTING*	
LENTIL	*8 HRS SOAKING*	*12 HRS TO 3 DAYS SPROUTING*	

1.

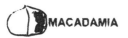 MACADAMIA *DOES NOT SPROUT*

MILLET *TO 3 DAYS SPROUTING*

 MUNG *TO 5 DAYS SPROUTING*

OATS *TO 3 DAYS SPROUTING*

 PECAN *DOES NOT SPROUT*

PEPITA *TO 2 DAYS SPROUTING*

PINENUT *DOES NOT SPROUT*

PISTACHIO *DOES NOT SPROUT*

QUINOA *TO 3 DAYS SPROUTING*

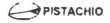 RICE *TO 5 DAYS SPROUTING*

SESAME *3 DAYS SPROUTING*

SPELT + RYE *TO 3 DAYS SPROUTING*

 SUNFLOWER *TO 3 DAYS SPROUTING*

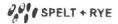 WALNUT *DOES NOT SPROUT*

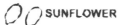 WHEAT *TO 3 DAYS SPROUTING* **119**

WORKS CITED

Arbour, Gilles. *Are Buckwheat Greens Toxic?* Townsend Letter for Doctors and Patients, December 2004

"Alfalfa." *Wikipedia: The Free Encyclopedia.* Wikimedia Foundation, Inc. Retrieved June 1 2014 from http://en.wikipedia.org/wiki/Alfalfa

Bairoch A. *The ENZYME database in 2000.* Nucleic Acids Res 28 (1): 304–5, 2000

Benzie, I. *Evolution of dietary antioxidants.* Comparative Biochemistry and Physiology 136 (1): 113–26, 2003

Bolander, FF. *Vitamins: not just for enzymes.* Curr Opin Investing Drugs 7 (10): 912–5, 2006. Retrieved May 20 2014 from www.ncbi.nlm.nih.gov/pubmed/17086936

Combs, Gerald F. *The Vitamins: Fundamental Aspects in Nutrition and Health.* Elsevier, 2008

Duke SO. *Overview of herbicide mechanisms of action.* Environmental Health Perspective #87: 263–71, 1990

Fallon, Sally and Mary G. Enig PhD. *Nourishing Traditions.* Warsaw: New Trends, 2000

Forbes, RM, HM Parker and JW Erdman Jr. *Effects of dietary phytate, calcium and magnesium levels on zinc bioavailability to rats.* The Journal of nutrition 114 (8): 1421–5, 1984

Foster, S. and J. A. Duke. *A Field Guide to Medicinal Plants. Eastern and Central N. America.* Peterson Field Guides, 1999

Helweg, Richard. *The Complete Guide to Growing and Using Sprouts: Everything You Needed to Know Explained Simply, Including Recipes.* Ocala: Atlantic Publishing Company, 2011

Howell, Edward. *Enzyme Nutrition.* Penguin, 1985. John Hopkins Medical Institutions. *Cancer Protection compound Abundant In broccoli Sprouts, John Hopkins Scientists Find.* Science Daily, 19 September 1997. Retrieved July 12 2014 from www.sciencedaily.com/release/1997/09/970919062654

Mercola, Dr. Joseph. *Broccoli-Sprout Beverage Helps Detoxify Environmental Pollutants.* Retrieved June 30 2014 from http://articles.mercola.com/sites/articles/archive/2014/06/30/broccoli-sprout-detox.aspx

Nelson, David L. and Michael M. Cox. *Lehninger Principles of Biochemistry, Third Edition* (3 Har/Com ed.). W. H. Freeman. p.1200, 2000. Organicfacts.net. *Health Benefits of Chlorophyll.* Retrieved July 10 2014 from http://www.organicfacts.net/health-benefits/other/health-benefits-of-chlorophyll.html

Peary, Warren and William Peavy, *Ph.D. Natural Toxins in Sprouted Seeds: Separating Myth from Reality.* Retrieved June 2, 2014 from chetday.com/sprouttoxins.html

Price, Weston A. *Nutrition and Physical Degeneration.* Price-Pottenger Nutrition Foundation: 8th edition, page 249, 2008

Reeves, Pat. *Minerals and Trace Elements In Sprouts.* Retrieved June 15 2014 from http://www.foodalive.org/articles/minerals_sprouts.htm

Shipard, Isabell. *How Can I Grow and Use Sprouts as Living Food?* David Stewart, 2005

Suzuki, U and, T. Shimamura. *Active constituent of rice grits preventing bird polyneuritis.* Tokyo: Kagaku Kaishi 32: 4–7; 144–146; 335–358, 1911

Szekely, Edmond Bordeaux. *The Essene Gospel of Peace: Book One.* International Biogenic Society, 1981

RESOURCES

www.sproutpeople.org – *A great source for info, seeds and equipment.*

www.sprouting.com – *Mumm's seeds offers many organic seeds, information and equipment*

www.sproutamo.com – *Home and travel sprouters for sale, a personal favorite.*

www.westonaprice.org – *Foundation with aim of promoting unbiased nutritional information and challenging politically correct diet assumptions.*

www.pfaf.org – *Plants for a Future database. Detailed and accurate information on many useful plants.*

www.essentialeating.com – *Producer and supplier of sprouted flours*

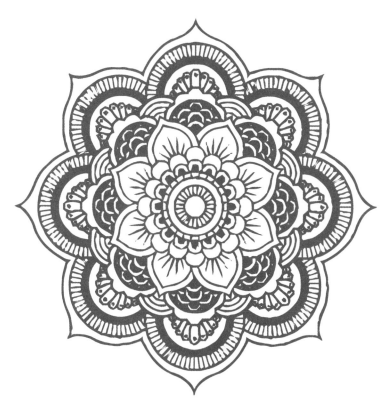

Sprout fresh life
Share the bounty
Eat peace

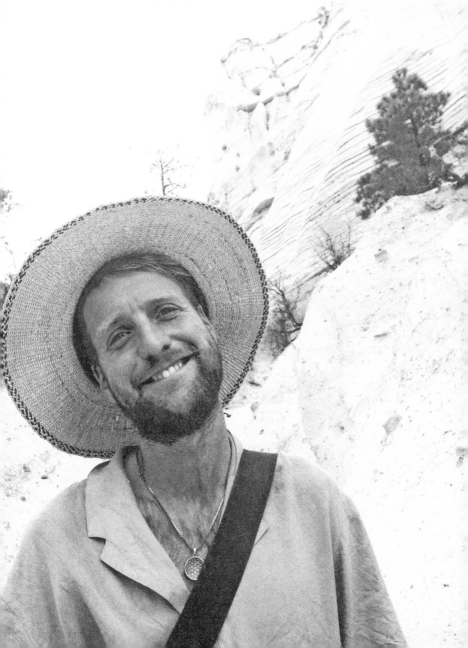

ABOUT THE AUTHOR

IAN GIESBRECHT, also known as Ini, has traveled around the world learning about many different food cultures. Originally from Canada, he currently lives on an eighteen-acre homestead bordering Caney Creek in Ozark County in southern Missouri, where he and his partner Wren are developing and cultivating an edible and medicinal perennial ecosystem.

SUBSCRIBE TO EVERYTHING WE PUBLISH!

Do you love what Microcosm publishes?

Do you want us to publish more great stuff?

Would you like to receive each new title as it's published?

Subscribe as a BFF to our new titles and we'll mail them all to you as they are released!

$10-30/mo, pay what you can afford. Include your t-shirt size and month/date of birthday for a possible surprise! Subscription begins the month after it is purchased.

microcosmpublishing.com/bff

...AND HELP US GROW YOUR SMALL WORLD!

Read more about the Food Revolution:

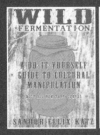
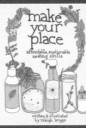
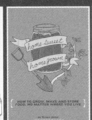
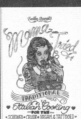
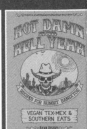